WEED
ALL ABOUT IT

A guide to growing, rolling, smoking,
and eating your green

DANNY MALLO

DOG 'n' BONE

WARNING: The serving quantities provided are suggestions only and will vary depending on the strength of the canna-butter/oil/milk and your personal tolerance levels.

This edition published in 2022 by Dog 'n' Bone Books
an imprint of Ryland Peters & Small Ltd
341 E 116th St   New York, NY 10029

Previously published in 2018

www.rylandpeters.com

10 9 8 7 6 5 4 3 2 1

Text © Danny Mallo 2018
Design © Dog 'n' Bone Books 2018

A CIP catalog record for this book is available from the Library of Congress.

ISBN: 978 1 912983 59 9

Printed in China

Editor: Clare Sayer
Design concept: Wide Open Studios
Designer: Jerry Goldie
Style illustration: John Riordan
Step illustration: Dan Prange

Thanks to the following for the images on pages 53–5:
Aphid: Alvesgaspar; Fungus Gnat: James Lindsey at Ecology of Commanster; Spotted Spider Mite: J. Holopainen; Thrip: OpenCage; White Fly: Gaucho; Leaf Miner: N3v3rl4nd

CONTENTS

– Part One –
GROW IT
INTRODUCTION

WARNING: GROWING WEED IS HIGHLY ADDICTIVE!

It is well known that smoking and eating cannabis is not addictive. What most people don't realize is that growing it is incredibly so. The moment you germinate that first little seed you will be hooked for life. As a hobby, it's very easy and surprisingly inexpensive to get into, plus it's also hugely rewarding; for less than you would typically spend on an ounce or two of weed you can build a basic indoor setup capable of yielding a pound or more in just a few months.

This book aims to make growing weed as easy as possible by presenting all the essential information in a way that even the most stoned mind can understand. At first some of the charts and the scientific stuff might seem like a lot to take in (especially if you've had a smoke before you get started!), but don't panic, everything is more simple than it might appear at first. Just follow the advice here and you'll soon achieve great results. There will be problems and disappointments along the way, but you will learn from them. Growing weed is very much a case of the more you put in (both in time and money) the more you get out. Fortunately, once you start growing you won't be able to stop!

As well as growing weed, this book will show you how to harvest your crop, make very potent hash, and make canna-butter/oil, which can be used in the recipes for some cannabis-infused culinary delights (see pages 128–141). So get your gardening gloves and chef's hat at the ready and give growing and cooking weed a try.

A BRIEF HISTORY

If you thought weed was just about getting stoned with your mates, you'd be wrong—there's a lot more to it than that...

Mankind's relationship with cannabis can be traced back about ten millennia to the end of the last ice age. This was an era known as the Neolithic Revolution—a time when people abandoned their nomadic lifestyle in favor of settling in one place where the focus was on farming rather than hunting and gathering. Around this time people were migrating into northern Asia from Africa. Luckily for us, this happened to be the home of the cannabis plant, and people were quick to make the most of this new miracle crop. Its versatility and ease of cultivation would make it one of the most important substances and most widely grown crops in human history.

Many cultures have used cannabis for manufacturing everything from rope, textiles, and paper to fuel, food, and even building materials. Of course, our ancestors also made the most of its medicinal and curative effects. It has been widely used throughout the ages for recreation, human bonding, and spiritual enlightenment. Although the industrial and medicinal use of cannabis has been greatly suppressed over the last century, many people are now rediscovering its many benefits.

It has been estimated that over 50,000 products can be manufactured from the cannabis plant, including building composites and plastics. The chemicals in cannabis can treat over 250 diseases and illnesses plus a long list of other ailments, making it a potential treatment for more conditions than any other substance. Its potential is so great that some believe it could actually stop wars, save the environment, boost economies, and improve the general health and wellbeing of humankind. So next time you're having a smoke, raise a joint in appreciation of 10,000 years of stoner history.

SATIVA, INDICA, AND RUDERALIS

So, what actually is it that you've been grinding up and rolling in your joints all these years? The first person to classify weed officially was Carolus Linnaeus, the Swedish botanist who devised the modern system for naming species. In 1753, using samples of European hemp that was widely cultivated at the time, Linnaeus named the plant Cannabis sativa L., "sativa" coming from the Latin word for "cultivated" and the "L" standing for Linnaeus (one of the conventions of the naming system). He considered it to be monotypic (having just one species) and believed it had originated in northern India. However, research in the 1930s by the Russian botanist Nicolai Vavilov identified it as originating in the Samarkand area north of Afghanistan and the Hindu Kush mountains.

In 1785 the French biologist Jean-Baptiste de Lamarck suggested that it was actually polytypic (having more than one species). His studies revealed differences between the European hemp and samples he had collected on his travels through India (a bit like many backpackers do today!) These plants varied enough to be classed as a distinct separate species, which he named Cannabis indica Lam. ("indica" representing its Indian heritage).

In 1924, almost 150 years after Lamarck's discovery, the Russian botanist D.E. Janichevsky was studying feral cannabis along the Volga River in Western Siberia and concluded that there was actually a third species. He called it Cannabis ruderalis Janisch., from the Latin word "rudus," meaning rubble—ruderal species of plants being those that first emerge from freshly disturbed ground.

How to tell cannabis plants apart by leaf shape

SATIVA

INDICA

RUDERALIS

In 1976, Canadian botanist Ernest Small and American taxonomist Arthur Cronquist suggested that the divergence between indicas and sativas was a result of human selection and cultivation, sativa being well suited to fiber and seed production and indica being used primarily for drug production.

This was backed up in studies also from the 1970s, by professors William Emboden and Loran Anderson, and Harvard botanist Richard E. Schultes. They concluded that there were indeed physical traits sufficiently different for cannabis to be categorized into the three separate species. The more widespread sativas, growing tall and sparingly branched with narrow leaflets, were normally found in warm lowland regions. Indicas, being shorter and bushier with wider leaflets, were adapted to cooler climates and highland regions, while the branchless ruderalis, being the shortest of the three, was found growing wild in Europe and central Asia.

You might think, "Why is this important to me?" Well, my green-fingered apprentice, read on...

How to tell cannabis plants apart by shape and size

SATIVA

INDICA

RUDERALIS

THE SCIENCE

Cannabis is a highly versatile and adaptable annual flowering herb capable of thriving at altitudes of up to 8,000 feet (2,400m). It has a life cycle of three to six months and can grow at a rate of 6in (15cm) a day (although 1–2in/2–5cm is typical). Some varieties can mature as small as 12in (30cm) while others may stretch to 20 feet (6m) and beyond—about the size of your average two-story house.

Cannabis plants are dioecious, which means they will be either male or female—male flowers produce pollen and females make the seeds. Both male and female plants have glands that secrete a sticky resin, although the females produce much more. These glands, called "trichomes," are most prevalent on the flowers, which if left unpollinated will continue to swell and grow, forming large columns of resin-coated buds known as "colas." This resin contains chemicals such as Delta-9-Tetrahydrocannabinol (THC) and Cannabidiol (CBD), known collectively as "cannabinoids." These chemicals are responsible for the mental and physical effects that a user experiences. In other words, they are the stuff that gets you baked.

These cannabinoids work by interacting with cannabinoid receptors in the brain and indirectly increasing the levels of a neurotransmitter called dopamine (neurotransmitters are chemicals that occur naturally in the brain and are used to transmit information and send messages to the body). When dopamine is released, it makes a person feel good, and at these increased levels it produces the psychoactive (or mashed) effects that you are no doubt familiar with.

The type of cannabis you use can have a significant impact on the effect experienced. THC produces the uplifting, cerebral "high" that a user experiences, while higher CBD levels can lead to an increase in the physically relaxing "stoned" feeling (a characteristic favored by many medicinal users). Additionally, higher levels of another cannabinoid called cannabinol (CBN) can lead to increased uneasiness, anxiety, and disorientation. If you've ever thrown a whitey, you'll be all too familiar with these effects.

Indica strains were developed throughout history primarily for cannabis's medicinal benefits. As such they now typically have higher proportions of CBD than sativa strains. This makes indica strains generally more relaxing, providing a "body stone" ideal for chilling out in the evening, while sativas give more of an energetic and euphoric high—perfect for daytime smoking when you need to get stuff done.

The colorful world of weed

MODERN CULTIVATION

You've had the history and science lessons, now it's time to learn how weed and the culture surrounding it has evolved.

Before the 1960s the vast majority, if not all, of cannabis consumed in Western Europe and North America was imported and generally differentiated by its country of origin. In the early 1960s large-scale importation of weed and hash was rapidly increasing. Most of the weed smuggled at that time was produced from sativa strains and contained seeds. However, these seeds gave people the opportunity to experiment with growing their own, especially in tropical areas such as Florida and California. By the late 1960s certain strains, such as Panama Red and Acapulco Gold, had gained legendary status.

In the early 1970s growers began producing weed without seeds, known as sinsemilla, from the Spanish sin meaning "without" and semilla meaning "seeds." This was achieved by removing male plants to prevent the female plants from being pollinated. This causes the females to put all their energy into making big, swollen, resin-rich flower buds instead of seeds—resulting in a higher-grade product.

By the mid-1970s sinsemilla was the leading type of domestically grown cannabis. Cultivators soon began developing strains suited for indoor growing under artificial lights, allowing them to control the heat and light and in turn increase the potency and yield of their plants. Cross-pollination then led to selective breeding of plants for particular traits such as flavor, smell, or color. Further crossbreeding and inbreeding eventually resulted in some of the famous sativa strains of the 1970s, such as Purple Haze, Maui Wowie, and Eden Gold.

The mid- to late 1970s also saw the introduction of indica strains to Europe and North America from Central Asia and the Middle East. These shorter, bushier, and earlier-maturing plants soon became popular as they were easier to hide, often more potent, and usually more cost-effective for the grower than their sativa cousins. It wasn't long before breeders were cross-pollinating sativa and indica strains to create plants with the bushy, early-maturing, and potent traits of the indica but with the more uplifting high of the sativa strains.

By the 1980s cultivation of sinsemilla had become more common, and the vast majority of plants grown had traces of both sativa and indica genetics. Owing to political pressure on US growers and a more relaxed view in the Netherlands, the reins of the cannabis-breeding industry were passed from the Californians to the Dutch. With advances in growing techniques and a better understanding of the plant, the Dutch breeders went on to make some of the most famous strains known today, and established themselves as the leaders in cannabis cultivation. Although it must be noted that almost all the Dutch varieties owe their genetic heritage to a handful of the North American strains grown in the 1960s and 1970s.

In the mid-1990s, the attitude of the Dutch authorities began to change, and stricter limits were put in place for the coffee shops. Meanwhile, the opposite was happening across the pond. In 1996, California enacted Proposition 215, allowing the medicinal use of cannabis, and this was followed over the next few years with similar laws in Oregon, Maine, Nevada, and Colorado.

The twenty-first century saw increasing pressure on the Dutch, with many coffee shops being shut down. However, the pro-cannabis sentiment in the US was increasing. Laws for medicinal use or decriminalization were introduced across numerous states, and in 2012 recreational use was legalized in Colorado and Washington, with other states to follow. This dramatic overhaul of the legal landscape meant that the US was now back in the driving seat, propelling the science and business of cannabis forward to become the multi-billion-dollar industry that it always had the potential to be.

PLANT GENDER

And now it's time for a bit of sex education. As mentioned earlier, cannabis plants are dioecious, meaning that they are either male or female. However there are occasionally plants that are monoecious, bearing both male and female flowers, known as hermaphrodites. Sometimes female plants can even become hermaphroditic when subjected to stress, such as from a lighting failure or physical damage, so be sure to treat your ladies with respect.

So, how can you tell if your plant is a guy or a girl? Well, at around six to eight weeks old a plant will begin to show pre-flowers, which look like single regular flowers, consisting of a small green pod (calyx). These can be found at the branch internodes (the point where the branch meets the stem) just behind the leaf stipule (the small spur at the base of the branch). Female pre-flowers can be determined by a pair of white hair-like pistils emerging from the calyx, while male pre-flowers do not develop these.

How to identify the sex of cannabis pre-flowers

PISTILS

STIPULE

CALYX

PRE-FLOWERS

FEMALE

MALE

When genders have been established, remove any males from the crop. This stops females from becoming pollinated, allowing them to grow large, swollen flower buds. Once pre-flowering has started, plants are mature enough to be triggered into flowering by switching the light cycle (see page 18). You can keep them in a vegetative state for longer if you wish, but never switch before pre-flowering as the stress can produce hermaphrodites, which can pollinate themselves and other plants in a grow room. Once the light cycle is changed, growth slows and things start to get interesting, as flowering will be visible within a couple of weeks. Male plants are taller with fewer leaves, and tend to flower before females. Male flowers resemble miniature bunches of bananas or coconuts that hang from the plant and release a cloud of pollen, which is carried by the wind to the females.

Female flowers consist of a calyx, containing an ovule out of which emerges a pair of pistils. As she matures, more calyxes develop and swell into large, densely packed buds covered in THC, and the pistils darken to orange, red, or brown. If a female is pollinated, bud growth slows up and just one seed will develop in each calyx. The seeds contain almost no THC, which is why you don't want plants to be pollinated.

How to identify the sex of cannabis flowers

STAMINATE
FLORAL BUD

STAMINATE
CALYX

STAMEN

FEMALE   **MALE**

FEMINIZED SEEDS

Regular cannabis seeds will typically produce a 50/50 ratio of male to female plants. For some growers, especially those with a restricted grow space, growing double the number of plants that they ultimately want is impractical. Fortunately it is now possible to get feminized seeds, which produce female plants 90 percent or more of the time.

AUTOFLOWERING

Not everyone has access to huge, isolated outhouses in which to grow massive trees of weed. For many of us space is at a premium, particularly when you need to keep your crop under wraps. In such circumstances time is usually an issue too: the quicker you can harvest your plants, the less chance of your grow operation being discovered. That's where "autoflowering" plants come in handy.

Sativa and indica strains of cannabis are triggered into flowering when the amount of light and dark in a day reaches a certain level, around 12 hours of each. However, the shorter, lower-strength ruderalis varieties (see page 6) begin to flower at a certain age, regardless of light levels, and this trait has been successfully exploited in the development of autoflowering strains.

In the 1970s the Canadian botanist Ernest Small tried crossing ruderalis with more potent strains to make a plant that was compact and autoflowering, but still packed a punch. Unfortunately, the results were only partially successful—while compact and autoflowering, the plant contained only intermediate levels of THC. In the 1980s, Small's early work inspired Australian-born Nevil Schoenmakers, the "father of Dutch seed banks," to experiment with crossing ruderalis with more potent strains such as Skunk #1 and Northern Lights, but again the potency wasn't what he had hoped for.

Thankfully for stealth growers, in the late 1990s the true champion of ruderalis announced himself to the world: a Canadian known only as the Joint Doctor. While living on a farm in Quebec, the Doctor was given a cannabis seed by a Mexican friend, Antonio, who had been cultivating cannabis for many years. The seed was from a strain called Mexican Rudy, one that stayed short and flowered very early but was of medium potency. It is believed that it had been produced at an American university during the 1970s by crossing Mexican cannabis with Russian ruderalis (hence the name Mexican Rudy).

The Joint Doctor grew the Mexican Rudy and proceeded to cross it with other strains: first a cross with Northern Lights, then the resulting offspring crossed with a William's Wonder clone. This hybrid, initially dubbed William's Automatic, would go on to be known famously as Lowryder. This strain matured automatically at no more than 12 inches (30cm) and in less than 60 days from seed. Further crossbreeding of the Lowryder has now led to autoflowering strains that are as potent as many of the top traditional varieties. It is now even possible to get feminized autoflowering seeds, which provide the benefits of small plants, a quick harvest, and no unwanted males. What more could you ask for?

THAT'S DOPE: where to buy seeds

Cannabis seeds are available from seed banks, many of which can be found online. It is said that the first seed bank was started in California in the 1960s by a group called the Sacred Seed Collective. In 1985, a member called David Watson (AKA Skunk Man Sam) moved to Amsterdam, taking with him seeds of some legendary strains. He soon met three breeders, to whom he gave the seeds: Ben Dronkers, Eddie Reekeder, and Nevil Schoenmaekers, owner of the Seed Bank of Holland. Over the next decade they crossbred the seeds and produced some of the most famous strains around. Eddie went on to start the Flying Dutchmen Seed Bank and Ben the Sensi Seed Club. In 1991, Ben bought Nevil's company and formed the Sensi Seed Bank, then in 2006 he bought the Flying Dutchmen, giving the Sensi Seed Bank one of the best catalogs of weed strains available today.

INDOOR GROWING

Now you're familiar with the background of this amazing plant, it's finally time to start planning your grow room. But before you start setting things up, it's worth considering the following factors:

Soil or Hydroponics: This is the first decision you need to make. The type of setup will have an impact on the grow room you choose. If using hydroponics, consider any extra space needed to accommodate reservoirs and other equipment (see page 24).

Space: A grow room should be a self-contained space adequate for the number of plants you plan on growing. You might have an entire room available or just a small cupboard under the stairs—both will do the job perfectly well. Specially designed grow tents (right) are a good shout; these handy units come in a range of sizes and have built-in vents and fittings for all your equipment.

Giving your plants plenty of space is vital; they need to be able to grow freely with room around them for airflow and light penetration. An ideal grow space should be at least 6 feet (1.8m) tall and allow at least 1ft2 (30cm2) of space per plant, although the more the better. You can successfully grow in a tiny space, just consider the various methods of training (see page 48) or using autoflowering varieties (see page 14), which can mature at just 1 foot (30cm).

Light: You want light to be able to reach all around your plants, so cover the walls with a reflective material such as Mylar® or simply paint the walls white. Do not use aluminum foil, as this can heat up and burn plants. Light escaping from a grow room is one way of getting busted, so ensure there are no leakages. It is also important that no light can get into your grow room during dark hours. See page 18 for more information on lighting.

Heat: This can be a problem in small spaces. Make sure the surrounding area is not prone to extremes in temperature. When the lights go out the temperature can decrease dramatically, and cold temperatures are as much of a threat as high ones. Cops have also been known to use heat maps to detect grow operations. So maintaining a typical room temperature (68–79°F/20–26°C) in the surrounding area is important, especially if growing in a loft. See page 38 for more about temperature.

Air Supply and Odor Control: To control heat and keep your plants happy, a grow room needs a supply of fresh air and a route for the old air to escape through. For fairly small spaces, a room with a window should be fine. Your area should also be as airtight as possible to contain any odors—you don't want the wrong people smelling out your stash. See page 20 for more about ventilation.

Water: Like me and you, plants get thirsty and want a good drink from time to time. You will need constant access to water and a way to dispose of any unwanted liquids, so make sure these aren't too far away. Nobody wants to be lugging heavy buckets up three flights of stairs each time your plants need watering. Also, if using hydroponics, you will need to take precautions to avoid any floods or spills.

Noise: Fans echoing through ducting can get noisy and get you caught (plus the sound will do your head in!), so locate your grow area away from anywhere it could easily be heard. Acoustic ducting and ventilation silencers can be used to reduce any noise.

Cleanliness: Pests and diseases thrive in dirty conditions, so maintain a high level of cleanliness both in your grow room and in the surrounding area. Do not have carpets or other surfaces in your grow area that can't be washed clean.

Safety: Water and electricity do not mix! Any grow area has lots of both, so be sensible. Keeping all electrical equipment and cables high up is a good way to avoid accidents.

Security: People get caught because of laziness, complacency, or greed. Don't cut corners, make assumptions, or take unnecessary risks. Always think one step ahead, be constantly vigilant, and do not trust anyone.

LIGHTING

Nope, this isn't about the age-old issue of where you last saw that box of matches. This is a key element of growing weed that you don't want to be in the dark about.

With the exception of autoflowering strains, cannabis plants are photoperiodic, which means they begin to flower when the balance of light and dark reaches around 12 hours of each. At the start of your grow, use an electric plug timer to give your plants 18 hours of light per day to keep them in their vegetative growth stage.

When they finally get to the size you want, trigger the flowering stage by switching the light cycle to 12/12. (During flowering, a plant will usually double in size, so bear in mind how much space you have in your grow area before reducing the hours of light.) Autoflowering strains should be given around 18–20 hours of light per day throughout the entire life cycle.

> The color spectrum of the light will have an impact on your plants. The blue spectrum simulates the light of spring and is suited to vegetative growth, while the red spectrum, simulating summer light, is better for the flowering stage.

TYPES OF LIGHTING

High Intensity Discharge (HID): These are the most common lights used for growing weed. They are either metal halide (MH) or high-pressure sodium (HPS), intended for the vegetative and flowering stages respectively owing to the spectrum of light emitted.

When buying HID bulbs you will also need to buy a ballast (which limits the current supplied), a contactor (used for safe automatic switching), and a reflector or hood. HID bulbs produce a lot of heat, so air-cooled hoods are often used as these have their own independent ventilation. HID lights are available in a range of sizes—use a minimum of 30W/ft2 for vegetative growth and 50W for flowering. The table opposite details the different wattages of HID bulbs available.

How to choose HID lighting for your grow room

Wattage	Coverage Area	Distance from Plants
150W	2ft^2 (0.6m^2)	4–11in (10–28cm)
250W	2–2.5ft^2 (0.6–0.8m^2)	5–13in (13–33cm)
400W	3–3.5ft^2 (0.9–1m^2)	6–19in (15–48cm)
600W	3.5–4ft^2 (1–1.2m^2)	8–25in (20–64cm)
1000W	4–5ft^2 (1.2–1.5m^2)	10–31in (26–79cm)

Compact Fluorescent Light (CFL): CFLs use less electricity than HID lights but are not as effective, with the light only being useful up to a distance of 2 feet (60cm). However, it is still possible to get decent results with CFLs, especially with short plants in small grow spaces. CFLs don't give out as much heat as HID lights, so they can be positioned closer to the plants and require considerably less ventilation. They are often used for seedlings and clones, so if you start with CFLs and move onto HID lights you will still be able to make use of them.

It is recommended to have a minimum of 45W/ft2 for vegetative growth and 65W/ft2 for flowering. The best for vegetative growth are the "daylight" spectrum bulbs rated as 6500k, while the "warm white" (2700k) bulbs are best suited to flowering.

Light-emitting Diode (LED): The most efficient grow lighting, producing the least heat and lasting the longest of all grow lights. Unfortunately they are very expensive, and there are lots of badly made LED setups on the market, so be careful when making a purchase.

> You should hang the lights in your grow room in a way that allows them to be raised as your plants grow—chains or specially designed light hangings are ideal.

VENTILATION

Now it's time to take a deep breath and get ready for the exciting topic that is ventilation. Well, I say exciting, it's not quite as fun as rolling up a joint from your first crop of home grown, but setting up a good ventilation system is vital for a number of reasons: plants absorb carbon dioxide for photosynthesis; fresh air reduces humidity that can encourage diseases and pests; the movement caused by airflow helps to strengthen the plants; and air replenishment is needed to maintain optimal temperatures. Finally, ventilation can also reduce that telltale smell, so all in all it's a pretty important element to think about.

The basic principle for setting up a grow-room ventilation system is that there should be an intake of cool, fresh air and a route to exhaust old, warm air. Because hot air rises, the exhaust should be near the top of your grow room and the intake at the bottom. An inline fan is used to blow the air out of the exhaust (known as an active exhaust). Although fans can be used for the intake, it's generally okay just to have an opening (known as a passive intake). The intake should be a little smaller than the exhaust to create negative pressure in the room and prevent odors escaping through any other gaps.

Pushing air through a carbon filter

HOT AIR PULLED OUT

HOT AIR BLOWN OUT OF FILTER

PASSIVE INTAKE

COLD AIR PULLED IN

The air expelled by the fan can be pushed through a carbon filter to remove any odor. Alternatively, it can be pulled through the filter and then expelled through the fan. Inline fans are rated by the amount of air they pass in a given time, measured as cubic feet per minute (cfm) or meters cubed per hour (m3/h). Ideally, the fan should replace the air in your room once every minute, although hot grow rooms, particularly those with HID lights, may need five or more exchanges per minute to keep the temperature under control.

Pulling air through a carbon filter

CARBON FILTER FAN

HOT AIR BLOWN OUT

GROW TENT

HOT AIR PULLED INTO FILTER

CLIP FAN

PASSIVE INTAKE

COLD AIR PULLED IN

In order to calculate your required cfm rating, work out the volume of your room by multiplying the length by width by height (in feet). So the volume of a room 2 feet long by 2 feet wide by 6 feet high would be 2 x 2 x 6 = 24 cubic feet. Therefore you need a fan rated at 24cfm or above. To calculate the m3/h rating calculate the volume of your grow room (in meters) and multiply by 60.

Other factors will also have an impact on the airflow. For example, bends in ducting will reduce the flow by around 5–10 percent. If adding a carbon filter, you should increase the fan rating by about 25 percent. In addition to the ventilation fan, it is also necessary to have one or more fans circulating the air inside the grow room. Clip-on desk fans should do the job.

For very small stealth grows, inline fans and carbon filters may not always be needed. PC fans can be a great alternative for small projects. If you are still concerned about the smell, there are tubs of odor-absorbing gel available from grow shops and online that can be placed in a grow room.

GROWING MEDIUMS

All growing mediums have their advantages and disadvantages. Some people argue that the only way to go is hydro, while others swear on their mother's life that soil grows are the best. My advice: try them all yourself to see which best fits your needs.

Soil is the most common and easily accessible for beginners, but as you hone your skills, you will possibly find that the flexibility and control offered by the hydroponic substances make them a better choice.

Soil: Soil can consist of rock, sand, clay, moss, and other organic material. It also contains microorganisms to break down organic material and are essential in providing soil with its life-giving properties. Most commercial soils will have added fertilizers. When buying soils you need to consider the NPK values (see page 44). Use seedling compost for young plants, as they are particularly sensitive to nutrient burn.

Soil is a smart choice for first-timers—it's cheap and fairly easy to maintain, and there is much less need to test the pH than with a hydroponic setup. On the downside, soil encourages pests and diseases, and it is more difficult to flush if there is a nutritional or chemical problem. Drainage is another common problem, so be careful not to under- or overwater. If using soil, mix it with about 25 percent perlite, to help with water retention and drainage.

> Never use soil from your garden, unless you are planting outside, as it contains pests and diseases. Even if you are growing outside, you are better off filling a hole with fresh soil or a mixture of old and new.

Coco Coir: This is an eco-friendly by-product of coconut processing. It is highly aerated, encouraging roots to grow to their full potential, and is completely inert, meaning that it has no nutritional properties. It can be used in hydroponic setups or as you would soil. Coco coir has naturally occurring rooting hormones to promote healthy root growth, and offers higher resistance to fungal infections and root disease than other mediums. Coco coir does tend to absorb calcium and magnesium, so use a cal/mag supplement.

Rockwool: This is a lightweight, inert hydroponic medium with excellent water-retention properties. Resembling loft insulation, it is made by spinning molten rock into fibers, which are then formed into cubes and slabs of various sizes. A good size cube for seedlings and cuttings is 1½in (36mm), before moving on to another growing medium or larger cubes. It has a high pH, so before use it should be soaked in water with a pH of 5.6 for several hours.

Expanded Clay Pebbles: This is an ecologically sustainable growing medium, made from porous clay pebbles that are ideal for hydroponic grows. They are inert and pH neutral, but wash them before use to remove dust. They are pricier than other mediums, but can be reused, saving you money in the long run.

Perlite: Made by heat-expanding volcanic glass, these highly absorbent granules are inert and pH neutral. They are usually combined with other growing mediums to aid water retention and drainage, but can also be used on their own. They contain a lot of dust, so rinse well before use and never use in a recovery hydroponic system (one that recycles the excess fluids) in case it gets drawn into the pump. Vermiculite is similar to perlite and can be used instead.

HYDROPONIC BASICS

For newbie growers, hydroponics might look more suited to a NASA laboratory than a closet grow room, but it's actually a lot simpler than it may seem at first.

Hydroponic setups use a nutrient solution in water and, instead of soil, plants are grown in a water-retaining medium (see page 22). The first benefit of hydroponics is that the roots are provided with a lot of oxygen, often with the aid of an air pump. Secondly, the nutrients are more abundant than in soil and under conditions that make them easier to absorb, resulting in larger plants that grow faster. Hydroponic solutions are also less susceptible to infection from pests and diseases. Below are the six main types of hydroponic system.

Wick System:
This is the simplest method. Nutrient solution is drawn up a wick from a reservoir and into the growing medium. An air pump, connected to an air stone, is put into the reservoir to aerate the solution.

GROWING MEDIUM

GROW TRAY

RESERVOIR

WICK

AIR PUMP

AIR STONE

DRIP MANIFOLD

DRIP LINE

OVERFLOW DRAIN PIPE

NUTRIENT PUMP

Drip System:
A timer-controlled pump in the reservoir pumps nutrient solution up to a drip line, dripping it onto the base of the plants. Some systems collect the excess run-off solution back into the reservoir—this is known as a recovery system.

FLOATING
PLATFORM

NET POT

Deep Water Culture
(DWC): A deep reservoir is filled with nutrient solution and net pots are floated on the surface using a foam raft, or are suspended just above the solution, with only the roots outside the pots being submerged (see DIY DWC on page 26).

Ebb and Flow
(aka Flood and Drain):
A submerged water pump, controlled by a timer, pumps nutrient solution from the reservoir into the grow tray. Once the tray is flooded the pump switches off and the solution drains back into the reservoir. This is repeated every few hours or so.

GROWING
MEDIUM

OVERFLOW
DRAIN PIPE

WATER
PUMP

GROW
TUBE

Nutrient Film Technique
(NFT): The nutrient solution is pumped into a downward-sloping tube so that a shallow film of solution flows down it. The plants are suspended through the tube with the roots hanging down, touching the passing solution.

WATER
PUMP

Aeroponic: In this system the roots are suspended in air and misted with a spray of nutrient solution every couple of minutes.

MISTING
NOZZLE

WATER
PUMP

DIY DEEP-WATER CULTURE SYSTEM

So you want to try hydroponics? Well, a homemade DWC system is the perfect place to start. This guide explains how to make a bucket system to fit a single plant, but the same principles, along with a larger container, can be used to make a multiple plant system. You'll be swimming in green in no time.

You will need:

- 4–5 gallon (20–25 liter) bucket with lid (ideally black or a dark color to prevent algae)
- Net pot: approximately 5in (14cm)
- Sharp knife
- Power drill with ¾in (19mm) and ³⁄₁₆in (5mm) drill bits
- Rubber grommet: ½in (13mm) inside; ¾in (19mm) outside
- ½in (13mm) 90-degree elbow connector
- ½in (13mm) clear tubing (ideally green or blue to prevent algae)
- Cable tie
- Strong glue or a hot glue gun
- Air stone
- ¼in (6mm) airline tubing (length will vary depending on distance from bucket to pump)
- Air pump rated at a minimum of 65gal/hr (300l/hr)
- Permanent marker pen

1 Mark out a circle in the center of the bucket lid, slightly smaller than the diameter of the net pot, and cut it out with a sharp knife. Make sure the pot fits snugly in the hole. It's best to cut the hole a little too small first and then adjust it, rather than making it too big.

2 Using the ¾in (19mm) drill bit, make a hole in the side of the bucket about ¾in (19mm) from the bottom. Insert the rubber grommet into the hole and insert the 90-degree elbow connector into the grommet. Using the ³⁄₁₆in (5mm) bit, drill a hole in the side of the bucket about 2in (50mm) from the top.

3 Cut a length of the ½in (13mm) tubing approximately 3in (75mm) shorter than the height of the bucket, and push one end onto the elbow connector. This will act as your water level indicator and a way to refill and empty the reservoir. Using the knife, make two small holes vertically in line with the elbow connector, approximately 4in (100mm) from the top of the bucket and about ½in (13mm) apart. Feed the cable tie through the holes to make a loop, which will keep the indicator tube held upright.

4 Using the glue, stick the air stone to the bottom of the bucket. Connect the airline tubing and pass it through the ³⁄₁₆in (5mm) hole (made in step 2). Connect the other end of the tubing to the air pump.

5 Now it's time to work out the water levels. Fill the bucket with water so that, when the lid is put on the bucket, the water level reaches about ½in (13mm) below the bottom of the net pot. Mark this level on the ½in (13mm) tubing with a permanent marker pen. This will be the level required when the roots have eventually grown through the net pot. Now add more water to the bucket so the water level reaches about ½in (13mm) above the bottom of the net pot. This will be the water level required before the roots have emerged.

6 Now, add your nutrients to the water, pot up your plant using clay pebbles, and switch on the air pump.

7 Use an EC meter to check the reservoir strength regularly and top up as needed (see page 46). Because the plant roots will be submerged in the nutrient solution, it is important that an optimum reservoir temperature of around 60-70°F (16-21°C) is maintained. You should also regularly check the pH (see page 40) and adjust as required, aiming for a pH of around 5.8.

DIY EBB AND FLOW HYDROPONIC SYSTEM

Now you've got your feet wet with a DWC system, here's something a bit more advanced to try. The ebb and flow system uses a water pump, but is still a simple project. The steps explain how to make a two-plant system, but could easily be adapted for any number.

You will need:

- A dark-colored plastic storage/tote box with lid: approximately 20 gallons (100 liters) capacity
- ½in (13mm) clear tubing (ideally green or blue to prevent algae)
- Rubber grommet: ½in (13mm) inside; ¾in (19mm) outside
- ½in (13mm) 90-degree elbow connector
- Cable tie
- Plastic tray roughly the same length and width as the storage box but about a third as high (plastic cement-mixing trays work well, or you can cut down a second box)
- Power drill with 1¼in (32mm) hole saw and a ⅜in (10mm) drill bit, and a ¾in (19mm) drill bit
- ¾in (19mm) ebb and flow fitting set
- 20in (50cm) length of black irrigation tubing with ½in (13mm) inner diameter
- Submersible water pump rated at approximately 120gal/hr (600l/hr)
- Air stone

- ¼in (6mm) airline tubing (length will vary depending on distance from bucket to pump)
- Air pump rated at a minimum of 65gal/hr (300l/hr)
- Electrical plug timer
- 2 net pots: approximately 5in (14cm)
- Expanded clay pebbles

1 Use the clear tubing, grommet, elbow connector, and cable tie to make a level indicator tube as shown for the deep-water culture project (page 26).

2 Cut two 1¼in (32mm) holes in the center of the plastic tray. Place the tray on top of the box lid, taking care to line it up so it is central. Mark the holes onto the tray before drilling them out too. With the ¾in (19mm) drill bit, cut another hole in the lid as shown.

3 Fit the ebb and flow fittings (left) into the holes of the tray.

4 Attach the irrigation tubing to the water pump outlet and put it into the storage box. Trim the tubing so that the pump can sit on the bottom of the box with the tubing just meeting the lid when it is put on. Position the air stone inside the box.

5 Put the tray on top of the lid, lining up the fittings through the lid holes. Now connect the irrigation tubing to the underside port of the inflow tube.

6 Connect the air stone to the airline. Run the airline and the water pump cable through the small hole in the lid (drilled in step 2). Connect the other end of the airline to the air pump.

7 Half fill the storage box with water. Do this in 1 gallon (5 liter) increments and mark the levels on the indicator tube for future reference.

8 Turn on the water pump. It will begin pumping water from the reservoir into the grow tray. When the water reaches the level of the overflow pipe it drains back into the reservoir. Use the timer to set the water pump to come on for 15 minutes, three times per day during the plant's light hours. Throughout the grow you may need to adjust the timing, especially in hot temperatures, when the growing medium will dry out quicker. The air pump should stay on permanently.

9 Plant your seedlings or clones in your chosen growing medium (see page 22) in the net pots and position them in the grow tray. Fill the rest of the tray with the clay pebbles to stop light getting to the roots and to support the weight of the plants.

10 Use an EC meter to check the reservoir strength regularly, and top up as needed (see page 46). Unlike with DWC systems, reservoir temperature is not as much of a concern in an ebb and flow setup. You should still regularly check the pH (see page 40) and adjust as required, aiming for a pH of around 5.8. Before you know it you'll have a pair of bud-smothered plants ready to be chopped down and enjoyed.

GERMINATING SEEDS

Some seeds are lazy little bastards and need a bit of encouragement. Rather than putting them straight into your growing medium, give your seeds a kickstart by sprouting them first using the method below.

You will need:
- A small container with a lid, such as the plastic boxes from takeout restaurants
- Some paper towel
- A bottle of distilled or mineral water

1 Fold a few sheets of paper towel so they will fit into the container, and pour on some water so the towel becomes thoroughly wet but not drenched. Place the seeds on top of the towel and fold the wet paper over the top of them.

2 Put the lid on the container and put it somewhere dark at a temperature of around 70-88°F (21-31°C). Check occasionally to make sure the paper towel hasn't dried out. After 24-72 hours the seeds will crack open and a white sprout called a radicle will pop out. This is the root or taproot.

3a If growing in soil, take a small pot approximately 4in (10cm) in diameter and fill it with a 50/50 mixture of seedling compost and either perlite or vermiculite. Water the soil so that it is wet but not soaking. Use a pencil or similar to poke a hole about twice as deep as the length of the seed.

3b If you plan to grow hydroponically it's best to use rockwool starter cubes. Before use, soak the cubes for several hours in water adjusted to pH 5.5 (see page 40), then shake them to remove any excess water. Use a pencil or similar to open up the hole (or create a hole if there's not a pre-made one).

4 Gently place the seed into the hole with the sprout facing downward and cover with a thin layer of medium. Some growers choose not to pre-germinate, and instead put the unsprouted seed directly into the growing medium. If you choose this option ensure that you plant the seed with its pointed end facing down.

5 Place the pot or rockwool cube inside a propagator with a transparent cover. This will act like a small greenhouse keeping the air inside moist and warm—perfect for encouraging seedlings to grow. Put the propagator under suitable seedling lights (CFL lighting is ideal) for 18 hours per day, aiming for a temperature of around 70-77°F (21-25°C). To reduce the risk of mold, occasionally lift up the propagator cover to provide fresh air.

6 After a day or two the little seedling will finally make its way out of the soil, revealing a pair of tiny round leaves called cotyledons. As soon as it comes through, remove the pot or cube from the propagator. Leaving seedlings in humid conditions for too long can cause rotting or a fungal infection called "damping off." Keep the seedlings under the seedling lights for a few days before moving to more powerful lights. Cannabis seeds can be expensive, though, so turn the page for a way to get weed plants for free.

CLONING

This might evoke images of mad scientists, Dolly the Sheep, or a shit Michael Keaton film that I saw when I was mashed, but really it's just an old technique to replicate plants, commonly known as taking cuttings. All cannabis seeds are different, each producing plants with their own distinct characteristics. However, by taking a cutting, a plant can be cloned, creating a second plant with the same genetic makeup as the first. As such, it will have the same physical tendencies too (including gender, size, and flowering time). Therefore, many growers select plants from their crops that exhibit desirable characteristics and use them to make genetically identical clones. This method also eliminates unwanted males and is usually faster than starting from seed.

Cuttings should only ever be taken from a plant while it is in its vegetative stage (i.e. not while flowering), and cuttings taken from lower down are easier to root than those from high up. Also, nitrogen stored in the mother plant can inhibit rooting of the clones, so it's advisable to flush it first for around a week prior to taking cuttings (see page 40).

HOW TO TAKE CUTTINGS

You will need:

- Small pot of soil and perlite or rockwool cube
- Sharp blade
- Sterilizing agent/rubbing alcohol

- Rooting hormone (ideally a gel variety, but powder can be used)
- Propagator
- Spray bottle filled with dechlorinated water

1 If growing in soil, fill a small pot with a 50/50 mixture of seedling compost and perlite, and water thoroughly. If growing hydroponically, use a rockwool cube soaked overnight in pH 5.5-adjusted nutrient solution at a strength of around 350ppm (see chart on page 47), and shake off any excess water before use. Use a pencil or similar to make a hole in your growing medium about 1in (25mm) deep.

2 Cut off a side shoot from the mother plant approximately 2-4in (5-10cm) long with a new growth tip and at least one leaf internode, two if possible (a leaf internode is where a leaf connects to the stem).

3 Sterilize the blade and use it to carefully slice off the lower petioles (leaf stems) flush with the main stem. Now cleanly cut through the stem at a 45-degree angle, approximately ¼in (6mm) below the previous cuts.

4 Immediately dip the stem into the rooting hormone, making sure it covers the cut parts of the stem. Get the stem into the rooting hormone as quickly as possible to avoid air entering the cut. Put the cutting into water if there's going to be a delay.

5 Now put the cutting into the soil or rockwool and gently pack down the medium around the stem, securing it in place. If the cutting has particularly large leaves you can trim them down slightly so the clone can focus its energy on rooting rather than supporting the extra vegetation.

6 Mist the inside of the propagator with water and place the cutting inside. Place it under suitable lighting for around 18 hours per day (CFL lighting is recommended). Every few hours, lift up the cover to supply fresh air. Until the cutting has grown roots it will be obtaining all its moisture through its leaves, so keep it humid and regularly mist with water.

7 After a week, remove the cutting from the propagator for an hour. If the cutting does not wilt, leave it out for another hour and check again. If it is okay then it probably has sufficient roots to support itself. If it wilts, spray it with water and put it back under the cover for another day before checking again. Once out of the propagator, keep the cutting under the CFL lighting for a few days before moving it to the more powerful HID lights.

POTTING UP

What's that? Pot? I'm afraid not that kind of "pot " just yet; we're talking about the type to put your seedlings in. Potting up is the process of growing a plant in a smaller container and increasing the size in stages, rather than planting directly into the final container, as this can slow down growth and increase the risk of pests and diseases.

Most growers re-pot their plants after about two weeks into 5–6in (125–150mm) pots. Next, when the roots have completely filled that pot (but are not potbound), they transplant to the final pot size—3 liters minimum but 11 liters is typical (6 liters for autoflowering strains). Use plastic containers rather than wood, metal, stone, or ceramic ones as they can contaminate the medium. When potting up to your final size in a soil grow, use square pots rather than round ones as they are more space-efficient.

Anytime a plant is re-potted it causes stress, which can stunt growth for a few days, so don't re-pot once flowering has started. Similarly, owing to the short life of autoflowering strains, it's best to go straight from the starter container to the final pot size.

You will need:

For soil:
- 5–6in (125–150mm) pot
- Soil and perlite
- Gravel or clay pebbles

For hydro:
- 5–6in (125–150mm) net pot and clay pebbles

OR
- Rockwool cube

1 When the seedling is approximately 4in (10cm) tall, with several leaves and plentiful root growth spreading to the edges of the pot, it is ready to be potted up.

2 If growing in soil add a layer of gravel or clay pebbles to the bottom of your new pot to aid drainage. Fill the rest with a mixture of one part perlite to three parts soil, gently pack it down, and water. Make a hole in the soil big enough to fit the small pot inside. Some growers choose to add a root stimulant to the hole at this stage.

3 Gently squeeze and tap the small pot containing the seedling so as to loosen the soil from the pot. Then place your hand on top of the soil with the seedling stem protruding between your middle and fourth fingers.

4 Carefully turn the plant upside-down so it is balanced on the hand holding it, and use the other hand to remove the pot.

5 Now cup the soil and root-mass in both hands, trying to prevent it from breaking apart, and lower it into the hole. Add any extra soil around it to fill the hole, gently pack it down, and tap the sides of the pot so that all the soil settles down inside.

6 If growing in rockwool cubes you should be able to insert the smaller cube into the pre-cut hole of the larger one.

7 If using a net pot of clay pebbles, place the small pot inside the larger one, ensuring there is a layer of pebbles around all sides of the small pot, including above and below.

TEMPERATURE
AND HUMIDITY

When it comes to temperature, weed plants are a bit like Goldilocks: one minute they are too hot, the next they are too cold. You'll have to keep your eye on that thermometer to make sure the climate in your grow room is just right. The optimum temperature for growing weed is around 70–85°F (20–30°C) when the lights are on and 62–72°F (17–22°C) when they are switched off. Young plants prefer warmer temperatures with relatively high humidity, but as they get older they become more tolerant to colder and drier conditions.

As a rule, colder temperatures slow down growth, especially below 60°F (15°C), while freezing temperatures can shock or kill a plant. Colder temperatures can also encourage some types of mold, especially when damp. Cannabis plants are fairly resistant to heat, but anything above 85°F (30°C) will slow down growth and temperatures exceeding 95°F (35°C) can cause damage. High temperatures can also encourage infection and nutrient burn owing to increased water transpiration.

The temperature difference between lights on and off should not be more than 10°C (5°C is ideal). So if it is 28°C (82°F) with the lights on it should not go below 18°C (64°F) when they are off. This temperature shift affects the internodal length, with a smaller difference resulting in more compact plants and denser buds. During the first 2–3 weeks of flowering, some growers increase the night-time temperature to match the daytime to limit the internodal growth as much as possible, before reducing the night-time temperature back to its original level.

Flowering is the time when temperature is crucial and should be kept relatively low to increase yield and bud size. Reducing the night temperature in the last few weeks of flowering (often while it's being flushed) can also bring out any purple, pink, or blue shades in the buds. During these last few weeks, use a dehumidifier to reduce humidity as much as possible to encourage increased resin production in these final days.

The best way to monitor heat and humidity is with a digital thermometer and hygrometer. The ventilation can then be used to control the conditions with a humidifier/dehumidifier being introduced if further control of the humidity is needed. All strains of cannabis will have varying preferences of temperature and humidity, and it really comes down to experimenting and finding out your own individual requirements. However, the following table will give you an idea of what to aim for at different stages of the grow:

Optimum conditions for different stages of growth

GROWTH STAGE	TEMPERATURE	RELATIVE HUMIDITY
Seedlings and Cuttings	70–77°F (21–25°C)	70–80%
Vegetative Stage	75–82°F (24–28°C)	50–80%
Flowering Stage	65–77°F (18–25°C)	40–50%

As well as the environmental temperature, hydroponic growers also need to monitor their reservoir temperature. The oxygen-retaining capability of water is reduced as it heats up, so maintaining the correct temperature is highly important in order to provide sufficient aeration to the roots. Ideally you want to aim for 65–75°F (18–20°C). As you can see from the following data, a ten-degree rise can greatly reduce the oxygen level:

RESERVOIR TEMPERATURE	DISSOLVED OXYGEN LEVEL
10°C (50°F)	13 parts per million (ppm)
20°C (68°F)	9–10ppm
30°C (86°F)	7ppm

PH

Sadly, pH doesn't stand for pot heads (where would you be on the scale from 1 to 14?), but instead is the measure of how alkaline or acidic a substance is. A scale of 1 to 14 is used, with 1 being the most acidic, 14 the most alkaline, and a pH of 7 being neutral.

A number of elements are needed by a plant for nutrition—such as nitrogen and potassium—which are obtained through its roots. These various elements are more easily absorbed at differing pH levels, and at some points they can't be absorbed at all, which is known as "nutrient lockout." When this happens, the plant will show signs of deficiency in that element, despite it actually being present.

pH is much less of an issue for soil growers than for those using hydroponics, because the organic matter in soil has natural pH-buffering capabilities. Those growing with pH-balanced soil and using organic nutrients will be unlikely to have any pH problems, and only really need to check if something does go wrong. To measure pH, you will need either a digital pH meter or a pH testing kit. However, these are only suitable for testing liquids, so if growing in soil test the pH of the nutrient solution prior to watering your plants and then test the pH of the "run-off" (the liquid that drains from the pot). The midway point between the two readings is the approximate soil pH.

If a plant is showing signs of nutrient lockout caused by incorrect pH, flush the plants with pure, pH-adjusted water. To do this when using soil, pour twice the volume of the plant pot of water through the soil, wait for five minutes, and repeat. Then feed with only water for a week. Hydroponic growers should drain their systems and replace with water only, before introducing nutrients again after a few days.

Because the different elements are more easily absorbed at varying pH levels, it is best to let your plants experience a varied pH range. For soil aim for a pH of around 6.5–7.0; hydroponic solutions should be around 5.5–6.0 (see tables opposite for a detailed list of optimum pH). You can see from the tables how nutrient availability is affected by pH.

Nutrient lockout charts

SOIL GROW

	NITROGEN	PHOSPHORUS	POTASSIUM	MAGNESIUM	CALCIUM	ZINC	IRON	SULPHUR	MANGANESE	BORON	COPPER	MOLYBDENUM
5.0												
5.1												
5.2												
5.3												
5.4												
5.5												
5.6												
5.7												
5.8												
5.9												
6.0												
6.1												
6.2												
6.3												
6.4												
6.5												
6.6												
6.7												
6.8												
6.9												
7.0												
7.1												
7.2												
7.3												
7.4												
7.5												
7.6												
7.7												
7.8												
7.9												
8.0												

HYDRO GROW

	NITROGEN	PHOSPHORUS	POTASSIUM	MAGNESIUM	CALCIUM	ZINC	IRON	SULPHUR	MANGANESE	BORON	COPPER	MOLYBDENUM
5.0												
5.1												
5.2												
5.3												
5.4												
5.5												
5.6												
5.7												
5.8												
5.9												
6.0												
6.1												
6.2												
6.3												
6.4												
6.5												
6.6												
6.7												
6.8												
6.9												
7.0												
7.1												
7.2												
7.3												
7.4												
7.5												
7.6												
7.7												
7.8												
7.9												
8.0												

NUTRIENT LOCKOUT   NUTRIENT BEST AVAILABLE

To use this chart, measure your pH, then look out for any orange boxes indicating elements that may be unavailable to your plant.

> Use products called "pH Up" and "pH Down" to adjust the pH. Don't stir too vigorously before testing, as the extra oxygen can raise the pH. Air pumps have a similar effect, and you should test the pH again after an hour to check for changes.

NUTRIENTS

Imagine going on a date with possibly the fussiest eater imaginable. Now imagine this date lasts for four months. That's what it's like trying to keep your weed plant fed and happy!

Cannabis plants need over 20 elements to grow. Carbon, hydrogen, and oxygen are absorbed from the air and water, while the rest, known as mineral nutrients, are added to the nutrient solution. The three primary nutrients, which are required in the greatest quantities, are nitrogen (N), to promote growth of leaves and vegetation; phosphorus (P), to encourage root and shoot growth; and potassium (K), to regulate water and nutrient movement, and increase flowering and hardiness. When buying plant food, the primary nutrient content (or N-P-K values) will be written on the packaging as three numbers, with each number representing the ratio of these elements.

The secondary nutrients, which are required in smaller amounts, are calcium (Ca) and magnesium (Mg). These are followed, in even smaller quantities, by the trace elements iron (Fe), sulfur (S), manganese (Mn), boron (B), molybdenum (Mo), zinc (Zn), and copper (Cu). Finally, other elements such as aluminum, chlorine, cobalt, iodine, selenium, silicon, sodium, and vanadium are also needed, but in trace amounts that are normally present as impurities in the water or other nutrient products.

Although general-purpose fertilizer can be used, feeds (both chemical and organic) specially designed for cultivating weed are better. Just be sure to follow the manufacturer's instructions.

As a plant grows, it requires the various elements in different amounts. For rooting and germination, high levels of phosphorus with less nitrogen and potassium are needed. During vegetative growth, cannabis plants need lots of nitrogen, plus plenty of phosphorus and potassium, whereas a flowering plant will need less nitrogen and more phosphorus and potassium. For this reason cannabis nutrients are usually labeled for either vegetative or flowering growth.

As well as the main vegetative and flowering nutrients, there are many other additives available, some more beneficial than others. Using just the main nutrients alone will give great results, but as you gain experience you will no doubt experiment with some of these other products and discover what works best for you.

You can tell if your plant is lacking a particular nutrient by visual signs such as the discoloring of leaves or stems. This can often be remedied by using extra feed containing the deficient element, but be careful not to be misled by nutrient lockout caused by an excess of another element (see page 41) or an incorrect pH (see page 40). Adding more nutrients in these cases can actually cause more problems. You can use the table on page 44 to diagnose a nutrient deficiency.

THAT'S DOPE: getting the munchies

Why, after a smoke, do you get the urge to stuff your face with food? It's down to something in the brain called the endocannabinoid system, which consists of naturally occuring cannabinoids and the receptors that they bind to. When your stomach is empty a cannabinoid tells the brain you are hungry by binding to specific receptors. THC is chemically similar to this cannabinoid and binds to these "hunger" receptors, tricking your brain into thinking you need food. It also interacts with receptors in the brain's olfactory bulb, intensifying your sense of taste and smell; as well as in the *nucleus accumbens*, boosting dopamine levels, which makes scoffing food feel so good.

NUTRIENT DEFICIENCIES AND DIAGNOSIS

SYMPTOMS	N	P	K	CA
Yellow Upper Leaves	No	No	No	No
Yellow Middle Leaves	No	No	No	No
Yellow Lower Leaves	Yes	Yes	Yes	No
Red Stems	Yes	Yes	Yes	No
Necrosis	No	No	Yes	No
Spots	No	No	No	No
Growing Shoots Die	No	No	No	No
White Leaf Tips	No	No	No	No
Stunted Growth	Yes	Yes	No	Yes
Deformed New Growth	No	Yes	No	No
Yellow Tips	No	No	No	No
Twisted Growth	No	No	No	No

Look out for any of the symptoms below: they may be caused by a nutrient deficiency or overfeeding. If your plants show such signs, use this table to identify what nutrients your plant may be lacking.

S	MG	FE	MN	B	MO	ZN	CU	OVER FERT.
Yes	No	Yes	No	No	No	No	No	No
No	No	No	No	No	Yes	No	No	No
No	Yes	No	No	No	No	No	No	No
No	Yes	No	No	No	No	No	No	No
No	Yes	No	Yes	Yes	No	No	Yes	No
No	No	No	Yes	No	No	No	No	No
No	No	No	No	Yes	No	No	No	No
No	Yes	No	No	No	No	Yes	No	No
No	No	No	No	No	No	No	No	No
No	No	No	No	No	No	No	No	No
No	No	No	No	No	No	No	No	Yes
No	No	No	No	Yes	No	No	No	No

WATERING PLANTS

Cannabis plants are snobs: they turn their leaves up at plain old tap water and instead want to drink something a bit more refined. The truth is, tap water can contain a few nasty chemicals, such as chlorine, that your plants won't appreciate, so be sure to dechlorinate it first. Products are available that do this, or simply leave water to stand for 2–3 days and the chlorine will evaporate. You should also establish the pH of your nutrient solution and adjust if necessary (see page 40).

SOIL GROWING

Cuttings and seedlings do not need feeding for the first couple of weeks; just give them water. After that, gradually move them onto the feeding schedule for your chosen nutrient range, ensuring it is one intended for soil use. Knowing when to water your plants is simple: if the pot feels light and the top few inches of soil is dry, water it. If the soil is damp under the surface or it still feels fairly heavy, then leave it a day or so. Overwatering can lead to problems, so make sure plants have ample drainage and are not left to stand in run-off liquid for too long.

Unless your nutrients say otherwise, do not change to flowering feed as soon as you switch to a flowering light cycle. Instead use the vegetative feed until growth has slowed and flowering has begun.

Once a month, give a feeding of just pure water to your plants. This reduces the risk of problems from nutrient build-up. Finally, two weeks before harvest, flush the plants by stopping the supply of nutrients and feeding them with water only until harvest (see page 56).

HYDROPONICS

A very weak nutrient solution can be used for seedlings and cuttings. After that, gradually move onto the schedule for your chosen nutrient range. As with soil growing, don't change to the flowering feed until flowering has begun. Finally, flush the plants one week before harvest.

Regularly check the pH of your reservoir and adjust as required (see page 40). You should also regularly check the nutrient concentration, known as the total dissolved solids (TDS), with an electrical conductivity (EC) meter. This gives the TDS measurement expressed in parts per million (ppm). Water evaporation and absorption by the plants will lower the reservoir water level and can raise the TDS. Top up the reservoir daily, with plain pH-balanced water to lower the TDS back to the desired level or 50 percent strength nutrient solution to raise it. Every two weeks completely drain the reservoir and fill it with a fresh batch of solution. The following shows the recommended TDS and pH levels throughout different stages of a hydroponic grow:

	INDICAS		SATIVAS	
	TDS	pH	TDS	pH
Seedlings/cuttings	300–400ppm	5.3–5.5	250–350ppm	5.3–5.5
Early vegetative	500–600ppm	5.3–5.6	300–500ppm	5.3–5.6
Middle vegetative	600–800ppm	5.4–5.6	500–700ppm	5.4–5.6
Late vegetative	800–1000ppm	5.5–5.7	700–900ppm	5.5–5.7
Early flowering	1000–1300ppm	5.5–5.7	1000–1100ppm	5.5–5.7
Middle flowering	1400–1600ppm	5.5–5.8	1100–1300ppm	5.5–5.8
Late flowering	1000–1100ppm	5.5–5.7	800–1000ppm	5.5–5.7
Ripening	300–500ppm	5.4–5.6	300–500ppm	5.4–5.6

Overfeeding is a common mistake growers make. It is better to give too little than too much—underfeeding may slow growth but overfeeding can be fatal. Healthy plants should generally be a bright shade of green, while very dark leaves are a possible sign of overfeeding. Similarly to lockout from incorrect pH (see page 41), overfeeding some nutrients can lead to others being locked out, giving the impression of a deficiency. Be careful not to confuse the two. To treat, flush the plants as described for a pH lockout (see page 40). The nutrients affected by an excess of other elements can be seen in the table below:

ELEMENT IN EXCESS	ELEMENT AFFECTED	ELEMENT IN EXCESS	ELEMENT AFFECTED
Nitrogen	Potassium, Calcium	Copper	Iron, Molybdenum, Manganese, Zinc
Potassium	Nitrogen, Calcium, Magnesium	Zinc	Iron, Manganese
Phosphorus	Zinc, Iron, Copper,	Molybdenum	Copper, Iron
Calcium	Boron, Magnesium, Phosphorus	Sodium	Potassium, Calcium, Magnesium
Magnesium	Calcium, Potassium	Aluminum	Phosphorus
Iron	Manganese	Ammonium Ion	Calcium, Copper
Manganese	Iron, Molybdenum, Magnesium	Sulfur	Molybdenum

TRAINING

What if I were to say to you that with just a little bit of extra effort and without the need for any magic potions, mystic incantations, or voodoo rituals, you could considerably improve your harvest? Well, my young pot padawan, I'm going to do exactly that.

Although you can grow weed plants wild and free, you may find that a little training can dramatically increase your yield or help control the size and shape of a plant. The main methods used are low stress training (LST) and high stress training (HST). The latter causes physical damage to the plant to get the desired results, so only use it during the vegetative stage, when there is time to recover. For the same reason, this method is not recommended for autoflowering strains.

HOW IT WORKS

Cannabis plants contain hormones called auxins that cause the growth of buds. These auxins are most concentrated at the top of the main central shoot that stretches up toward the light, known as the apical bud. As well as promoting bud growth, the auxins also inhibit bud growth elsewhere on the plant. Removing (or repositioning) the apical bud halts the inhibiting effect, increasing auxin levels elsewhere, resulting in multiple new apical buds.

HIGH STRESS TRAINING (HST) TECHNIQUES

Topping: This is used to increase yield and decrease height. The whole apical bud (or more of the plant) is cut away at a 45-degree angle, causing the two side shoots below to become new apical buds. Topping can be repeated on the new growth, resulting in the development of even more bud sites.

FIM CUT

TOPPING CUT

The FIM Method: The "F**k I Missed" method was stumbled upon by a grower who tried to top a plant, missed, and only removed part of the apical bud. This resulted in several new bud sites rather than the two achieved by topping. To FIM a plant, use sharp scissors to cut about 80 percent from the top of the apical bud. This can be repeated on any new growth.

Lollipopping: For this method of training, lower leaves and side shoots are removed. This does not increase the total yield but it will increase the size of your main buds, eliminate lower "popcorn" buds, and improve air circulation within the plant.

Super Cropping: This involves squeezing and bending the stem into a 90-degree angle, applying enough pressure that you feel a slight cracking in the stem and can fold it over like a kinked hose. This can be repeated on other suitable branches. Over time the bend will heal and the plant will produce auxins in other areas that are exposed to lots of light, resulting in bushy, bud-smothered plants.

STEM BENT AT 90 DEGREES

LOW STRESS TRAINING (LST) TECHNIQUES

Bending and Tying: Here, plants are trained to grow horizontally by bending and tying them down using wire or string. Any time the plant is tied down it will grow back toward the light, so regular bending and tying are needed. Like super cropping, this spreads auxin production along the stem, resulting in more bud sites.

Screen of Green (SCROG)*: This is similar to bending and tying, but the plant is grown beneath a wire screen. As the plant grows, it is bent down and tied to the screen, resulting in a dense, shallow canopy of buds. SCROG is usually combined with lollipopping and topping/FIMming.

* Don't confuse with Sea of Green (SOG), which is a method for growing lots of miniature plants packed together to create a dense but short layer of foliage.

PESTS AND DISEASES

As a weed smoker, your number one enemy was most likely to be the cops busting your sorry ass for lighting up in public. Don't get me wrong, the police are still to be avoided at all costs, but the biggest threat to your plants is now from a smaller, but just as irritating group: bugs, and their accomplices fungi and bacteria. These little bastards get everywhere, so be extra vigilant because prevention is always easier and more effective than treatment. If you do happen to get affected, I've recommended some chemical treatments in the following pages, which are available from garden centers, grow shops, or online.

Grow rooms and equipment should always be kept clean and tidy. Grow your plants at optimum temperatures in a contained space with ample ventilation. Never use equipment that was previously used outside unless it has been sterilized, don't reuse soil, and always sterilize reusable hydroponic mediums and other equipment between uses.

PESTS—IDENTIFYING AND TREATING

Aphids: Usually gray or black but can vary in color. They remain stationary while sucking nutritional liquid from any area of a plant. To make matters worse, while tucking into your precious crops these aphids exude a sticky honeydew, which attracts ants.

Physical Treatment: Remove small infestations from your plants by hand. Use sticky traps to catch aphids and other bugs.

Chemical Treatment: Insecticidal soap, pyrethrum (aerosol).

Fungus Gnats: The long-legged, winged adults are 2–4mm long, gray/black, and usually found toward the base of the plant as they like to lay their eggs in the soil. The 4–5mm-long larvae have clear bodies with black heads and eat through roots, which then causes fungal infection— another problem you have to deal with.

Physical Treatment: Encouraged by humidity and damp soil, so provide ample ventilation and do not overwater.

Chemical Treatment: Bacillus thuringiensis var. israelensis (Bti) for adult gnats. Neem oil or insecticidal soap soil drench to kill larvae.

Leaf Miner Maggots: Despite having a pretty cool name, these are tiny maggots that burrow through leaf matter. As they munch your plants, they leave behind a telltale white outline of their tunnel, so you know you've been messed with.

Physical Treatment: Crush the visible maggots inside their tunnels and remove severely infested leaves.

Chemical Treatment: Water plants with a 0.5 percent solution of neem oil.

Spider Mites: The most common pest for indoor growers, these tiny eight-legged critters live underneath the leaves and suck out liquid. Look out for the yellowish-white spots they leave stippled on the tops of the leaves. The two-spotted mite is most common, but red and yellow-white varieties are also found.

Physical Treatment: Treat small infestations by reducing temperature to 60°F (16°C) and blasting the mites off with cold water. Remove leaves with more than 50 percent damage. After infestation, fully clean the grow room with 5 percent bleach solution.

Chemical Treatment: Neem oil, pyrethrum, horticultural oil, or insecticidal soap. Spider-mite eggs hatch in 5–10 days, so use two or three applications at 5–10-day intervals to kill them all.

Thrips: Tiny winged insects about 1–1.5mm long. They tend to move in groups, making them easier to spot. Whitish-yellow specks are left behind on top of leaves, which can darken and crumble from lack of chlorophyll.

Physical Treatment: Manual removal is possible, but they can be difficult to catch.

Chemical Treatment: Pyrethrum or insecticidal soap sprayed 2–4 times at 5–10-day intervals.

White Flies: Can be detected by shaking a branch and seeing if they fly out from the leaves. Like mites, they suck from the plant, leaving behind white stipples and signs of diminished chlorophyll.

Physical Treatment: None.

Chemical Treatment: Spray with natural sprays, insecticidal soap, or pyrethrum. Before spraying remove any leaves with over 50 percent damage and then apply spray at 5–10-day intervals.

FUNGI, VIRUSES, AND BACTERIA

Botrytis, also known as gray mold, is a bluish-gray hairlike fungus that starts within the buds and can even affect harvested weed. To prevent it, keep buds dry, maintain less than 50 percent humidity, and provide sufficient ventilation. If harvested, fully dry and cure before storing (see page 56).

Downy mildew appears as whitish-yellow spots on top of leaves with bumps of mycelium spores opposite on the underside. Spreading rapidly, it causes a lack of vigor and slows growth with leaves turning yellow and dying.

Powdery mildew exhibits itself as little bumps on top of the leaves which develop into a pale, powdery coating. It can be prevented with the use of high light levels, low humidity, and a plentiful air supply.

Root rot causes roots to turn from white to brown. Leaves show signs of chlorophyll depletion followed by wilting and slowed growth. It is most common when roots are stood in un-aerated water for a long time.

Damping off (also known as Pythium wilt) is a fungal condition that is usually brought on by damp soil. It attacks seedlings and cuttings, causing them to lose girth, weaken, wilt, and die.

Viruses and bacteria can also attack cannabis plants. Signs include spots, blotches, or swirling patterns on leaves, sickly growth, yellowing, wilting, low yields, and death.

TREATING FUNGI, VIRUSES, AND BACTERIA

Remove any infected plants form the grow room. Bordeaux mixture is an effective treatment for many fungal conditions, but there are no biological or chemical treatments for viruses. Consuming infected weed can be bad for your health, so unfortunately, if a problem is too wide spread, you may need to destroy the whole plant.

HARVESTING, DRYING, AND CURING

Finally, at long last, the time you've been patiently waiting for has arrived. You've not been this excited since you were a kid waiting for Santa to show up on Christmas morning. So what are you waiting for? Clear the decks and get those scissors ready!

Cannabis plants are best harvested when their buds are at full ripeness, and there will be a window of 5–7 days in which to do this. Around 1–3 weeks before peak ripeness, a plant's growth will slow and its pistils will darken. But the best way to determine harvest time is by studying the trichomes with a pocket microscope. Their bulbous heads start off clear and colorless, ripening to a cloudy appearance as the THC increases, before turning amber or brown as the THC decays. By observing the rate of change, you can predict the optimum harvest and flush times. Harvest when all the trichomes are mostly cloudy, with a few starting to turn amber.

Tetrahydrocannabinol (THC) gives you the uplifting and cerebral "high" feeling, while another cannabinoid, called cannabidiol (CBD), provides the physically relaxing "stoned" feeling. As the trichomes darken, the THC decays and is converted into cannabinol (CBN), which causes the uneasy sensations a user may feel. When this change happens it makes the effects of the CBD more prominent. Some growers will delay harvest to get a more sedating weed, but this is really just a waste of THC. For a particular high, you should instead select a strain that naturally peaks at a certain level of THC and CBD.

Drying is important, as it causes decarboxylation (see page 129) and prevents weed from going moldy when it's stored. Once dried, the buds can be cured, evenly distributing any remaining moisture, enhancing taste, and increasing aroma.

HOW TO HARVEST, DRY, AND CURE

1 Flush your plants two weeks before harvest. Pour lots of water through the growing medium, wait a few minutes, and repeat. Feed with water only for the final weeks, stopping three days before harvest. Turn off all lights for the final 24 hours and reduce humidity to boost resin production. Harsh-tasting starches and sugars build up in foliage during the day but are stored in the roots at night, so cut the entire plant down or cut all the branches off while it is still in the dark.

2 Cut off any of the larger leaves that aren't covered in many trichomes.

3 Now cut or pull away all the sugar leaves—the smaller, more resinous ones. Remove them close to the stem or just trim them in line with the edge of the bud. Keep any trimmings, as they can be used for making hash (see pages 58–65) or for cooking (see pages 128–141).

4 The plants now need to be dried. This is usually done by hanging the branches on strings. For best results dry in the dark, with good ventilation, at 65–75°F (18–24°C) and a humidity of 45–55 percent. Check daily for mold. Some people prefer to swap stages 3 and 4, in what is known as a dry trim, as they find it improves taste and aroma.

5 It should take 5–7 days to dry enough for curing. Check by bending some stems: if the stem snaps it is ready to be cured, if it just flexes then it needs longer.

6 To cure the buds, cut them from the branches and put them in an airtight container. Any remaining moisture will evenly spread through the buds as they "sweat" in the container. Open for ten minutes every 4–5 hours so fresh air can get in. If they feel noticeably moist after sweating, leave them out for a few hours to crisp up.

7 After a couple of weeks the buds will have cured fully and will be ready for using or storing. They will be about 25 percent of their original weight. Store your weed in a refrigerator or a cool, dark place.

MAKING HASH

If your past experiences of hash were smoking a jet-black, rock-hard lump of something that tasted like burning rubber, then you're in for a treat. The often misunderstood world of hashish includes some of the purest, most potent forms of cannabis available, and is worlds apart from the cheap "rocky" that you smoked as a teenager and burnt holes in your parents' sofa.

Hash is made by separating the resin glands (trichomes) from the plant matter and binding them together, usually with heat and pressure. The heat and pressure also improve the potency through decarboxylation (see page 129). THC levels can be much higher in hash than in weed—up to 75 percent in hash and over 90 percent in hash oil, compared to 10–25 percent in weed. Hash making dates back thousands of years, rubbing and pressing being the two traditional techniques used. More recently the knowledge gained from these has been used to develop modern techniques such as ice-water and chemical extraction.

Rubbed hash is made by rubbing hands over fresh flower buds until they become coated with sticky resin, which is then collected up into a ball. As the ball is rubbed and warmed, the trichome heads burst and the THC oxidizes, giving the outside a dark brown or black color.

Pressed hash is produced by shaking dried buds over a mesh screen to separate off the trichomes, which are then pressed, sometimes with heat, to form a solid block. A finer mesh and briefer shaking will allow less vegetable matter through, resulting in a higher grade of hash.

Chemical extraction is used to make hash oil. The cannabis is mixed with a solvent, such as isopropyl alcohol or butane, which dissolves the resin. This solution is then filtered to remove the plant matter before the solvent is evaporated, leaving behind the hash, which can be viscous like oil or solid and shatterable like glass.

Ice-Water extraction is done by agitating weed in ice and water. The freezing temperature makes the trichomes brittle and easy to break away from the foliage. The oil-based trichomes will not dissolve in water and, being heavier than water, will sink, whereas the water-soluble material dissolves and the foliage floats. The trichomes can then be extracted and pressed into hash known as "iceolator." It is also called "bubble hash" because of the way it bubbles when a flame is held to it—the higher the purity, the more bubbles there are.

ICE-WATER EXTRACTION BAGS

In 1998 Mila Jansen, owner of the Pollinator Company in Amsterdam, invented a system for ice-water extraction using a specially designed set of bags which she called "Ice-O-Lator Bags." These consisted of three nylon bags with progressively smaller micron screens sewn into the bottom of each.

This method was then developed further by a Canadian known as Bubble Man. He added more bags with even finer screens (to separate the hash into more grades), and in 1999 he released his range, called Bubble Bags.

MAKING BUBBLE HASH WITH EXTRACTION BAGS

" If it don't bubble, it ain't worth the trouble," is a well-known saying among hash connoisseurs—and believe me, get these bags and you will be able to make some incredi-bubble hash. And the best part is that you can make it from the trimmings left over from harvest.

You will need:
- Set of ice-water extraction bags and appropriate size bucket
- Cold water
- Enough ice for your size of bags/bucket
- Broken up buds or trimmings that have been frozen while still fresh and undried
- Wooden spoon or handheld mixer with paddle attachment

- Metal spoon
- Pressing/blotting screen
- Thermometer

NB: Using as much weed as possible is not necessarily a good thing. The following maximum weights of weed are recommended for each size of bag:
1 gal—2oz/56g
5 gal—8oz/200g
20 gal—32oz/1000g

1 Place the bags inside each other so the bag with the largest screen size (the "work bag") is innermost and the screens get progressively smaller. Put the bags into the bucket.

2 Add some water and ice, half of the weed, more ice, the remaining weed, and top up with more ice and water. Stir so it is all mixed up and leave to stand until the temperature of the mixture gets to 39°F (4°C) or lower. Some people recommend using RO (reverse osmosis) water, a purer form of water that is available from aquarium shops.

3 Stir the mixture with the wooden spoon for 15 minutes to break the trichome heads from the weed. You can use a mixer but it will break up the weed more and lead to a lower-quality hash.

4 Let it sit for 15 minutes so that the trichome heads can settle through the screens. Then pull out the work bag, letting the water drain out. If any resin glands are stuck to the underside of the screen, rinse them off into the next bag.

5 Let the water sit for 30 minutes then pull out the second bag. You will see a layer of wet trichomes on the screen inside. Use the metal spoon to scrape it up and spread it onto the pressing screen.

6 Repeat for any remaining bags. Sandwich the resin within the screen and press out some of the moisture with paper towels. Leave out for a day or so to dry fully. It can then be crumbled and smoked straight away or pressed into a block.

Don't throw away the wet weed when you have finished. You can use it for a second ice-water extraction, a chemical extraction (see page 64), or making cannabis-infused ingredients (see page 130). Your plants will also love being fed the nutrient-rich leftover water.

MAKING BUBBLE HASH IN A JAR

If you're a bit of a cheapskate or have spent all your cash on growing equipment, channel your inner MacGyver and use an old jar and a coffee filter to mimic the effects of a bubble bag and make epic hash.

You will need:
- Large mason jar or similar
- Broken-up buds or trimmings that have been frozen while still fresh and undried
- Cold water
- Ice cubes
- Draining spoon and normal spoon
- Kitchen strainer (sieve) and a container for it to sit on
- 1 or 2 large paper coffee filters
- Baking tray or pressing/blotting screen

1 Fill the jar to about halfway with your weed, top up with ice cubes, and fill almost to the top with water.

2 Screw on the lid, shake for 10 minutes to break the trichome heads from the plant matter, then put in the fridge for 30 minutes.

3 The weed will have floated to the top and a layer of trichome heads will have settled to the bottom. Use the draining spoon to scoop out all the weed.

4 Place a coffee filter in the strainer (sieve), position it over the container, and drain the liquid through (use two filters to improve the purity).

5 The coffee filter will be coated in wet resin. Use a spoon to push it toward the center of the filter, then close it up and gently squeeze out some of the water.

6 Open out the filter, scrape up the hash and spread it onto the baking tray or screen. Leave to dry for a day or so. It can then be crumbled up to smoke straight away or pressed into a block.

Don't throw away the wet weed when you have finished. You can use it for a second ice-water extraction, a chemical extraction (see page 64) or making cannabis infused ingredients (see page 130). Your plants will also love being fed the nutrient rich leftover water.

MAKING ISO HASH

After drinking their own bodyweight in beer and then hitting a packed bong, many people find alcohol and weed don't mix very well. However, they are actually the perfect pairing when it comes to making ISO hash—a chemically extracted hash oil made using isopropyl alcohol. It is also called QWISO hash, which stands for quick wash isopropyl hash, "quick wash" referring to the short time the weed is in the alcohol.

You will need:

- Mason jar or similar
- Buds or trimmings that have been dried, crumbled, and frozen overnight
- Isopropyl alcohol, ideally 99 percent purity, but if not, use anything over 91 percent
- 2 kitchen strainers (sieves) and two containers that they will fit over
- Large paper coffee filters
- 1 or more flat-bottomed glass dishes
- Desk fan
- Single-sided razor blade or similar

1 Add your weed to the jar, cover with isopropyl alcohol, and leave to stand for 30 seconds.

2 Shake the jar vigorously for 30 seconds. Any longer and you will begin dissolving chlorophyll and other substances in the plant matter.

3 Place one of the strainers (sieves) over one of the containers and empty the jar into it. Put the strainer of wet weed to one side.

4 Place a coffee filter in the second strainer and position it over the second container (use two filters to improve the purity). Drain the alcohol through the filter.

5 Pour the filtered alcohol into a glass dish. Place by an open door or window with the fan positioned to blow any fumes outside. You can now do a second wash into another glass dish. It won't be as high grade as the first batch, but it will still make some great hash. You can even try doing a third one, too.

6 Leave the fan on until all the visible alcohol has evaporated. Then leave to stand for a further 24 hours to ensure it has been fully purged of alcohol. You will be left with a coating of sticky hash oil, which can be scraped up with the razor blade.

– Part Two –
ROLL IT
INTRODUCTION

Humans began cultivating cannabis in Asia around 10,000 years ago. Since then weed has been grown in almost every environment on the planet. Its versatility and ease of cultivation made it one of the most important and widely grown crops in history. Thanks to millennia of selective breeding, plus advanced crossbreeding programs since the 1960s, the cannabis plant has developed into countless varieties and today's weed aficionado is spoilt for choice.

This book is a celebration of both the variety now on offer and the huge role cannabis has played in bringing people together. Not only did it have a significant impact on the development of modern civilization, but many friendships have been forged by the hot, glowing embers of a joint. Unfortunately, as sociable as a joint may be, a standard "One-skin" doesn't go that far when shared. So for all those times when you've got a crew of smoking buddies to provide for (or if you just feel like getting extremely baked yourself!), hopefully the creations in this book will cater to your needs. Not only are some of them big enough to get a whole party high, but they're also definite conversation starters!

TOOLS OF
THE TRADE

In recent years, as recreational cannabis use has increased and its medicinal benefits are being rediscovered, head shops have appeared on most high streets and across the Internet selling a huge array of weed-related paraphernalia. From rolling papers and simple pipes to ornate glass bongs and sophisticated electronic vaporizers, these shops stock everything a stoner needs (except for the actual weed itself!). While many of the treasures found in these Aladdin's Caves of Cannabis are somewhat gimmicky and unnecessary, there are some that are essential for any master roller's collection!

ROLLING PAPERS

Papers are available in many colors, patterns, and flavors, but the two most important aspects are how it rolls and how it smokes. These depend on the size of the paper, its thickness, and what it's made from. When you first learn to roll you will probably find wide, thick papers are easier to handle and more forgiving. However, as you hone your skills, you will find the extra paper a hindrance and moving to narrower, thinner papers will lead to a superior roll and a better tasting spliff. Ultimately it's down to personal preference, but one of the most popular types of rolling paper amongst veterans are those made from pure, chlorine-free flax paper. These papers are very thin (almost transparent) but are incredibly strong.

No matter how good your papers are, sometimes you will still get a tear or a hole in your joint. If this happens, the gum strip can be cut from a rolling paper and used as a bandage. This technique is also used throughout the book for sealing the junctions of some larger joints. It's also possible to transfer the adhesiveness from one paper onto an area of another paper where there is no gum. This is particularly useful for joining papers end to end to create an extra-long paper (see page 78). Sometimes, though, especially when stoned, this can be a bit tricky and you may want to invest in a box of rip-style rolling papers. These contain a continuous length of rolling paper about 16 feet (5 meters) long!

GRINDER

The most common type, usually made from metal or plastic, consists of two cylindrical sections that join together with sharp teeth in between. Weed is put inside and the two halves turned, tearing the bud between the teeth into a fine consistency ideal for rolling.

TOBACCO

A big difference between European and US joint rollers is the use of tobacco as a mixer with weed. Europeans tend to use it, while Americans generally don't. For years, potheads on both sides of the pond have been disputing which is best. The answer is both are—they both get you high and that's the most important thing! There are, however, strong cases for both schools of thought: if your weed is slightly damp, dry tobacco can help a joint to stay alight; it makes a joint less potent (which is preferable to some who may find a pure joint too intense); and it also makes a bag of weed stretch further. On the downside, there are many health risks involved with tobacco use and smokers can easily become addicted to the nicotine.

TERMINOLOGY

Often in the United States, the word "joint" refers to a pure weed roll, while a "spliff" refers to a roll with a mix of weed and tobacco. In Europe (and this book) both words are interchangeable. Although weed can be smoked pure, hashish must be mixed with something else when rolled in a joint.

MIXING BOWL

One of the most annoying things to happen to a joint is for it to burn more down one side than the other, known as sideburning, running, or elvising. A way to avoid this, if using tobacco, is to mix your weed and tobacco first. Having some kind of small mixing bowl in your skinning-up box is much better than doing it in your hand or loose on the table top.

On a similar note: if you want to skin up outside, particularly if it is windy, take an extra baggie with you (the small grip-seal bags you tend to get weed in). Add your ground-up weed and tobacco to the baggie, breathe in a small amount of air to inflate it, seal it closed, shake it thoroughly, and then empty the smoking mix into your rolling paper.

CARD FOR ROACHES

In the US and some other parts of the world the roach refers to the butt of the joint that is left when most of it has been smoked. However, in Europe (and this book) it refers to a small piece of thin card that is rolled up and placed in the joint to act as a mouthpiece. In the US this is also known as a crutch or filter. Using a roach gives you something to hold, protects your lips from burning, prevents a build-up of tar and moisture, stops bits of the smoking mix from getting in your mouth, and means that less is wasted. Adding the roach before the roll can be tricky to begin with, but it will actually help to structure the joint and allow for a perfect fit.

How to Make a Standard Roach

Cut a piece of thin card, approximately ¾in (2cm) square. Any thin card or paper can be used but it is always best to use a piece that is unprinted, as some inks can give off toxic fumes when burned. This is where roach books are ideal; small booklets of card usually about ¾x2in (2x5cm)—the best are the plain, chlorine-free varieties. Cut the card with scissors rather than tearing it, as frayed edges can be prone to clogging up with tar. If you have to tear the card, quickly run a flame over the edges to burn away any fraying and leave a smooth finish.

Card and paper have a grain direction, just like wood, making them easier to roll in one direction than the other. If you try and roll them in the wrong direction they will keep folding at angles rather than creating a smooth curve. So first try to determine the grain and then roll accordingly between your fingers to form a small tube. Once rolled into a tube, widen one end ever so slightly, as this will help to form the conical shape of the joint.

How to make an "M" Roach

This technique is useful for making an extra-wide roach, as the folded card will prevent you from breathing in bits of smoking mix. It's also perfect for making a standard joint stand out from the crowd.

| Cut a piece of suitable card about twice as long as you would for a standard roach. | Fold back a small section a little narrower than the width of roach you want. | Fold this section back on itself an equal amount. | Then fold back one more time to form an "M" shape. | To finish, roll the remaining paper around the "M." |

To avoid getting a baggy section of joint next to the roach, skin up with about a third of the roach sticking out of the paper. When you've finished rolling, tap the roach in and it will help to compact the section of smoking mix next to it.

Other useful Items

- **PDT (pokey down thing):** Used to poke down the smoking mix in the end of your finished roll. It can be any thin instrument such as a matchstick or pen.
- **Scissors and a sharp knife:** For cutting roaches and papers.
- **A needle and tweezers:** Useful for unblocking roaches and any other fiddly jobs.
- **Lots of lighters and spare lighter fuel:** Have a few available, plus some extra fuel so you don't spend the night lighting joints off the stove top when your lighter runs out!
- **Spare rolling papers:** It's 2am, the shops are closed, and your mate utters those dreaded two words… "Last paper!" We've all been there; make sure it doesn't happen again.
- **Airtight jars/pots:** To stash your bud, keep it fresh, and contain the smell. Also, keep weed in a dark place—THC decomposes in sunlight.
- **Digital scales:** A sound investment for weed buyers who want to make sure a dealer provides the correct amount.
- **More spare rolling papers:** Stash these somewhere safe ready for the time when a drink gets knocked over, turning all your other skins into papier-mâché!

THE ROLLS:

STANDARD ONE-SKIN

The originator and trendsetter, this is the most important joint of them all! It doesn't matter if you are a rolling rookie or a battle-hardened rolling veteran, you must all pay homage to this the simplest and grandest of all joints. Scientists say this is the big bang of rolls! It paved the way for the other joints you will practice in this book, which all follow the same basic principles as the One-skin.

1 Take one king size rolling paper and lay it out flat with the gum at the top edge and facing toward you. If you want to use the whole paper, go straight to step 5.

2 A joint is typically rolled into a conical shape, so it's best to remove a strip of paper at a slight angle, making it narrower at the roach end. The amount of paper you tear off will depend on how fat you want your joint to be. Fold the bottom edge of the paper up so that the roach end almost touches the center crease and the other end is up about half as much. Run your finger along this fold so that it is well flattened.

3 Lick along this folded edge to moisten the paper, being careful not to wet the paper too much. Tear away the unwanted strip and run the torn edge gently through your fingertips to smooth off any fraying.

4 Fold this torn edge up to the top edge and crease along the new fold, then unfold the paper and lay it back out flat.

5 Add a roach to your preferred side (typically the left) and fill the rest with your smoking mix. Shape the mix so that it is narrower at the roach and wider toward the other end.

6 Carefully pick up the joint with each end between a thumb and forefinger. Roll the front and back sides of the paper up and down past each other, gently pinching and pressing the mixture more and more

into shape, while moving your thumbs and fingers back and forth along the length of the joint to smooth out any bumps.

7 Use your left hand to support the roach end, while using the other hand to move from left to right, shaping the mixture into a solid cone or baseball bat shape.

8 Now for the tricky part. Roll the front edge of the paper down in line with the top of the smoking mixture and use your left thumbnail to tuck the paper in behind the roach—make sure you tuck it in as tightly as possible.

9 With the roach end still pinched between your left thumb and forefinger, support the other end with your right thumb and middle finger, while using your right index finger to run along the length of the joint, tucking the rest of the paper in behind the smoking mixture. Lick along the gum and seal the joint.

10 Tap the roach end on a hard surface and use a pen or other suitable tool to poke down the mixture inside the joint. You may also find gently rolling the joint between your thumb and fingers while tapping and poking will help smooth it out and reduce any baggy air pockets. Any smoking mixture that has fallen out along the way can now be put back in the end of the joint and poked down.

11 Twist or pinch the end, give it another little tap for luck, sit back, and spark up!

THAT'S DOPE!

You are only allowed to move onto the next joint when you have learnt to appreciate the One-skin on a Zen-like level and can roll it one-handed with your eyes closed.

When you start learning to skin up you will probably find it easier to use a whole rolling paper. As you improve, you may find standard king size papers, even the slim variety, are too wide. Removing a strip of the paper will not only make it it easier to roll but will also give a smoother smoke.

SECRET AGENT

Your mission, should you choose to accept it: roll a joint that can go undercover in the real world. This master of disguise works by hollowing out a cigarette and replacing the tobacco with smoking mix and the filter with a roach. It may sound like a simple assignment but it takes years of classified training to succeed. Once you've rolled one, put on your best Sean Connery accent and tell your friends, "The namesh Bong, Jamesh Bong, would you like to ssshmoke a ssshpliff?"

1 Gently squeeze and roll the filter end of a cigarette between your thumb and index finger. You will feel the foam filter inside becoming loose from the surrounding cigarette paper and you should be able to pull the filter out (a needle or tweezers may help here).

2 Make a roach the same width and length as the filter section and insert this into the open end of the cigarette. You may want to make a second roach and put this inside the first so that the hole is not quite so big. Alternatively, make an "M" roach (see page 70).

3 Beginning at the tobacco end and working your way up, gently squeeze and roll the cigarette between your thumb and index finger so that all the tobacco falls out.

4 Now all that's left to do is add your smoking mix to the empty cigarette, a little at a time, while poking it down along the way until it is filled and packed in tightly.

Smoke this double-O doobie and it will leave you both shaken AND stirred.

PEN METHOD

So you've failed miserably at hand-rolling a spliff but are desperate for a joint! This technique might just save the day.

1 Lay out a king size rolling paper with the gum facing toward you, then place a pencil or pen along the center crease line. If you prefer a more traditional cone-shaped joint you could make a cone

out of paper or card, seal it with tape and use that instead of the pen. Alternatively, you can buy metal joint-shaped tools from most head shops that have been designed for this job.

2 Pick up the paper with the pen inside, roll down the front side of the paper, and tuck it in tightly behind the pen. Lick the gum strip and then roll the pen upward with your thumbs so that the paper is sealed around the pen like a paper tube.

3 Pull the pen out of the tube of rolling paper, leaving a section of pen inside, about the same length as a roach.

4 Fill the empty paper tube with smoking mix a little bit at a time, poking it down as you go.

5 Remove the pen and add a roach in its place. Give the joint a final tap, poke, and twist off the end.

TWO-SKIN

The Two-skin is perfect for when you only have small rolling papers, or when you want a joint that lasts twice as long. This is THE social joint: great for passing to mates and big enough to make sure there's some left for you when it comes back around. Mastering the technique for joining two papers end to end is an essential skill for any expert spliff-roller, and one which will be used throughout this book.

1 Take two king size or standard rolling papers. Lay them end to end with the right one overlapping the left one by approximately the width of the gum on your papers (usually around ¼in/5mm). On the left-hand paper lick the small section of gum that will be covered by the right-hand paper and seal the two together using just this small section of gum.

2 Take a third paper and fold it in half with its gum facing outward and moisten the gum by licking it. Place this paper in between the other two so that the moistened gum edge is lined up with the right side of the left-hand paper.

3 Flatten the right-hand paper down on top of this third paper so it is sandwiched between the two. After a couple of seconds (while the gum is still moist), slide out the third paper and smooth down the join between the other two papers. The adhesiveness from the gum on the third paper should have transferred to the others, sealing them together.

4 Add a roach and your smoking mixture. Move the smoking mixture into the rough cone shape that you want your joint to be.

5 Rolling a joint this length is fairly tricky and you will probably find you lose half the smoking mixture out one end while you are concentrating on the other. The trick here is to support the right end of the joint on your right hand, between your thumb and forefinger. At some stages you may need to rest it as far up as your wrist. As with the One-skin joint, roll the front and back sides of the papers up and down past each other, while pinching and pressing the mixture into shape. Then, keeping your left hand at the roach end, use your right hand to move up along the joint and smooth it out. Make sure the right end is being fully supported.

6 Bring the front edge of the paper down in line with the smoking mixture and use your left thumbnail to tuck the paper in behind the roach. Use your right forefinger to tuck the rest of the paper in behind the mixture, starting from the roach end and moving along. When you have managed to tuck the full length of the joint behind the mixture, lick the gum and seal the joint.

7 Give the roach end a tap, add any extra mixture that fell out during the roll, poke it all down, and twist off the end.

Twice as long and twice as strong, this jumbo joint will get you twice as stoned!

KING-L

ALL HAIL KING-L! ALL HAIL KING-L!
Get up off of your knees and find a place in court where you
can get your rolling gear out. If you want a big fat cone of
a doobie then the King-L is the joint for you. Perfect the
technique for this regal roll and it will show the realm that
you're no court jester.

1 Take two papers, typically king size; however, this method also works well when you only have small papers and fancy something a bit bigger and tastier than a small skin joint. Line them up at right angles with the gum strip at the top edge of the horizontal paper and at the left edge of the vertical paper. Lick the bottom half of the vertical paper and stick the two papers together.

2 Fold the bottom half up to extend the horizontal crease along the full width of the L. Depending on how big and fat you want your King-L to be, you may want to tear off the top right corner of the vertical paper as the extra paper can create a harsher smoke.

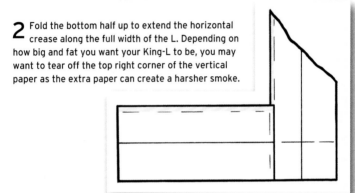

3 Add a roach to the left-hand side of the L and fill the rest with your smoking mix. Move the mix roughly into the shape you want, making the left side a little wider than the roach and the right side a few times wider.

4 Pick up the L and roll the paper between your fingers to shape the mix inside into a well-formed and dense cone shape. When rolled sufficiently, the mix should retain most of its own shape.

5 Using your left hand, carefully pull the front part of the paper down toward the top edge of the roach, while holding the shape of the mix together with your right hand. Use your left thumbnail to tuck the paper edge in behind the roach. Support the right end of the joint on your right hand and use your index finger to run along the top edge of the joint, tucking in the remainder of the paper. The flap of the vertical paper should be kept between the index and middle fingers for support.

6 Once the full length of the L is tucked in, lick the gummed edge of the horizontal paper and seal it down. Now lick the gummed edge of the flap on the vertical paper and wrap it around the joint.

7 Top up the joint with any smoking mixture left over and then give it a tap, poke, and twist. There you have it, a bifta fit for a king!

MAGNUM

You've got to ask yourself a question: do I feel lucky? Well, do ya punk? If you do, then maybe you're ready to put together this bad-guy beating, fast-car chasing, roof-top jumping mega joint; aka the Magnum. It's a King-L but rolled with the upright paper at an angle so that it makes the final piece even bigger! So big that you'll have to sign a waiver to get this hand-cannon out of precinct. Once you have got this technique down, you'll have to holster up and build a forearm of steel because this is one heavy piece of artillery... only the most badass, rule-breaking mavericks out there can handle it.

1 Lay out two king size rolling papers, as shown, with the paper behind making approximately a 135-degree angle to the front horizontal paper. Lick the gum strip on the paper behind, but only the section that is being covered by the horizontal paper, and stick the horizontal paper on top of it.

2 Using scissors or by carefully tearing, remove the bottom right corner of the horizontal paper along the line that has been stuck together. Also remove the bottom part of the paper behind in line with the bottom edge of the horizontal paper.

3 Add a roach to the left-hand side and fill the rest with your smoking mix. Use your fingers to move the mix roughly into the shape you want. Make the left side a little wider than the roach and the right side a few times wider. Pick up the Magnum and roll the paper between your fingers to shape the mix inside into a well-formed and dense cone shape. When rolled sufficiently, the mix should retain most of its own shape.

4 Using your left hand, carefully pull the front part of the paper down toward the top edge of the roach, while holding the shape of the mix together with your right hand. Use your left thumbnail to tuck the paper in behind the roach. Support the right end of the joint on your right hand and use your index finger to run along the top edge of the joint, tucking in the remainder of the paper. Support the flap of the angled paper between your index and middle fingers.

5 Once the full length of the paper is tucked in, lick the gummed edge of the horizontal paper and seal it down. Now lick the gummed edge of the flap on the vertical paper and wrap it around the joint. Top up the joint with some extra smoking mix, then give it a tap, poke, and twist.

Roll it, load it, and spin the cylinder, but be careful because, much like the recoil from a .44 Magnum, this joint kicks like a mule.

THREE-SKIN

As the saying goes, good things come in threes, and nowhere is this more true than when it comes to joints. So, all you aspiring spliff specialists, it's time for a Three-skin. This is the big bad wolf of the joint world: fat, mean, and, if you huff and puff on it for too long, your house might not get blown in but you'll certainly be pretty mashed. The structure is similar to a King-L but with an additional paper for extra width, allowing you to pack in a mountain of dope to get you, your mates, and the three little pigs nicely lean!

1 Flatten out three king size rolling papers, arranged as shown with the gum facing toward you.

2 Lick the gum on the bottom paper and stick it to the bottom edge of the top one. Now lick the gum on the remaining paper, but only as far along as will be needed to stick it to the other papers as shown.

3 This joint will be very wide, like a big Cuban cigar, so you'll need to place an extra large roach at the left end of the joint. Fill the rest of the paper with plenty of smoking mix.

4 Roll the Three-skin joint in much the same way as the King-L. Move the paper between your thumb and fingers to compress the mix into a well-formed solid shape. Then bring the front part down so that you can tuck the paper in behind the roach using your left thumbnail and the remaining paper with your right index finger.

5 Lick the gum, including the gum on the flap, and roll down. Roll and stroke between your fingers to make the joint nice and smooth, while giving it a gentle tap. Fill up any space in the end with some extra smoking mix and poke down until it's compressed and solid.

6 To prevent bits of smoking mix coming through the extra-wide roach, it is a good idea to make an additional roach, which can be put inside the first one. Alternatively, make an "M" roach (see page 70).

7 At this point it's probably a wise idea to call for some like-minded friends to come and help you enjoy this mammoth masterpiece!

ROLL REVERSAL

Also known as the "Flaming Backflip," this is the perfect joint for showing off with. It's much trickier to pull off than it may look, so mastering this technique is the sign of a true rolling professional and will be rewarded with nods of approval from those in the know.

This method ensures that only a single layer of paper encases the joint, which provides as clean and smooth a smoke as possible. Once rolled, it is party-trick time: light the excess paper like a fuse and watch the pot pyrotechnics. It's like all the fun of a fireworks display but without having to get your feet muddy!

1 Take one king size rolling paper and lay it down so the gum is facing down and away from you. Fold the paper back on itself along the center crease.

2 With the gum still along the bottom edge and facing out, add a roach and your smoking mix. Shape the joint roughly with your fingers so it is narrower by the roach and wider toward the other end.

3 Begin to roll it in the same way you would a normal One-skin joint, moving the paper back and forth and shaping the mix between your fingers. When the joint has been sufficiently shaped and the front of the paper brought

down in line with the top of the smoking mix, there are two possible options.

4 The gum can be licked and then tucked in behind the smoking mix, although this can be quite difficult to achieve.

5 The alternative is to tuck the gum strip in behind the smoking mix without licking it, using your left thumbnail for the roach end and your right index finger to tuck in the rest of the paper. The gum strip will now be covered by a layer of paper but not sealed. To seal the joint you need to lick through this outer layer of paper (only where there is gum strip behind) so that the gum strip also becomes moist and sticks to the outer layer. Be careful not to lick so much that the paper becomes sodden. You should now have what looks like a One-Skin joint but with an extra flap of paper protruding from one side.

6 The extra flap of paper can now be removed. While the licked area is still slightly moist you can tear it off. However, the sign of a true professional is to light the flap at the roach end. The flames will lick up the joint and burn away the excess paper.

THAT'S DOPE!

Extra kudos can be gained by getting the roach in your mouth quick enough to take a pull at the moment the flame reaches the tip so that it effortlessly lights the joint. Just be careful you don't set your hair on fire though!

DUTCH TULIP

Pack your bags, we're off to Amsterdam—the holy land for all European joint rollers. Home to some of the most potent skunk and hash you'll ever encounter, you'll want to take a piece of it home with you. "How?" I hear you ask. The answer is: "The Tulip." This botanical beauty is a dedication to the hazy times spent in the cannabis capital, and will make your eyes even redder than the famous lights themselves.

1 Take a piece of paper or thin card, about 4in (10cm) long and 1½in (4cm) wide.

2 Roll it between your fingers to form a slightly conical tube, approximately ³⁄₈in (8mm) in diameter at one end and ¼in (5mm) at the other. Wrap rolling papers around the tube to seal it closed. Alternatively, for an even more potent tulip, substitute this tube for a similar sized joint. However, if you're doing this, ensure the joint is a tight and solid roll that can support the weight of the tulip bud.

3 Now take two king size papers (or more if you want to make a bigger tulip). Lick the gum strip on one of the papers and stick it to the un-gummed bottom edge of the second paper to form a large rectangle. Use your hands to flatten it out.

4 Fold the bottom left corner of the rectangle up at a 45-degree angle so that the edge lines up with the bottom of the gum strip.

5 Without licking it, fold the gum strip down over the folded corner and run your finger along it to make a crease the full length of the paper. Fold back this crease slightly, lick the gum strip, and fold it back down so that it seals the folded corner.

6 Wait a couple of minutes for the gum to dry and then open the paper out. You should have something resembling a cone, with one side longer than the other.

7 Fill this cone with your smoking mix and pack it down to about ⅝in (15mm) from the top. Use a pencil to gently push the mix right into the tip of the cone (be careful not to push the pencil through the paper). Now push your paper tube just into the top of the mix.

8 Using your thumb and index finger, pinch the unfilled part of the cone around the paper tube so that the mix is tightly packed into the bulb.

9 Use scissors to cut the gum strips off two or three rolling papers and wrap them tightly around the pinched part of the tulip (a piece of string or thread can be used instead).

10 Bring the loose excess flap of paper over the bulb to form the leaves of the tulip. Now get ready to enjoy the full effect of a traditional Dutch delicacy!

SNAKE BITE

Fancy a joint with a bit of venom to it? Then get your lips
around a Snake Bite. Once you've smoked this slippery spliff,
you'll feel like you're in a snake charmer's trance and the only
known anti-venom is plenty of munchies! This reptilian reefer
combines three joints in one and will teach you the important
technique of using gum strips to seal any joins in your joints,
a skill that will be used throughout this book.

1 For this roll you will need one king size paper and two small papers, as well as a few extras for the gum strips.

2 Prepare the king size paper as you would for a standard One-skin (see page 72), with a roach at the left and smoking mix shaped ready for rolling. Do not put roaches in the two small papers, just fill them with smoking mix all the way along.

3 Roll the joints as you would normally, tapping and poking at the end. However, only twist the ends of the small joints. Leave about ⁵⁄₈in (15mm) of space at the end of the large joint and try not to compact the very last part too much. Insert the two small joints into the end of the large one.

4 Use scissors to cut the gum strips off a few extra rolling papers and stick one down through the middle of the two small joints as shown.

5 Take one or two more gum strips and wrap them around the joint, sealing it all together.

6 There it is: a snake that you want to be bitten by! Why not pack it full with some Durban Poison so its name is even more fitting?

CROSS JOINT

Made famous by Seth Rogen and James Franco in the brilliant stoner movie Pineapple Express. According to Franco's dope-dealing character, when lighting all three ends at the same time "the smoke converges, creating a trifecta of joint-smoking power." I don't know about that, but what I do know is this packs one hell of a punch and is more than capable of converting any non-believers of the weed! Just remember, you can't even light this thing on your own so make sure you've got a smoking buddy to help, not to mention three lighters!

1 Take one king size paper and one small paper, and lay them out with the gum facing up and toward you.

2 Add a large roach and plenty of smoking mix to the king size paper. You will need to make this joint large enough for the smaller joint to be able to pass through it. Prepare the small paper without a roach and with the smoking mix coming all the way to both ends.

3 Roll the large joint as you would a standard One-skin (see page 72) but don't compact the top half when you poke it or twist up the end too tightly; instead just pinch it closed. Roll the small joint so that it is uniform in diameter (not cone-shaped), poke both ends, and twist them.

4 Take a needle, toothpick, or similar sharp instrument and poke a hole through the large joint, about two-thirds of the way up. Slowly wiggle the needle around in a circular motion to widen the hole in the joint until it looks big enough for the small joint to fit through.

5 Start to push the small joint through the hole. When it is a little way through, use the needle to make a hole through the center of the small joint to allow the air to flow through. As before, wiggle the needle to open the hole up sufficiently.

6 Pull the small joint until it is halfway through the large one. Use scissors to cut the gum strips off three or four small papers and wrap one around each of the arms of the cross to seal the gaps.

7 Use the remaining gum strips to wrap all around the junction of the cross, sealing up any remaining gaps. Smoke one of these sacred spliffs and it will give a whole new meaning to "having a hot cross bun!"

DOUBLE BUBBLE

It may look and sound like a lollipop from your childhood but I can assure you that this is a much more complex and tasty joint than even Mr Wonka himself could have dreamed up. This is the Everlasting Gobstopper of tulip joints, made with extra papers to contain the whole heap of delicious, gooey, chocolaty smoking mix within*. However, once you've smoked this tasty treat, the room may soon be filled with dancing Oompa-Loompas singing annoying, toe-tapping songs you just can't stop humming along to.

1 Take a piece of paper or thin card, about 4in (10cm) long and 1½in (4cm) wide. Roll it between your fingers to form a slightly conical tube, approximately ³⁄₈in (8mm) in diameter at one end and ¼in (5mm) at the other. Wrap rolling papers around the tube to seal it closed.

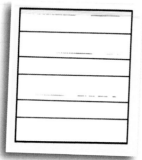

2 Construction of the Double Bubble is similar to that of the Dutch Tulip (see page 92) but with three king size rolling papers. Lick the gum strip on one of the papers and stick it to the ungummed bottom edge of the second paper. Repeat with the third paper and stick to the bottom edge of the first two.

3 Fold the bottom left corner of the rectangle up at a 45-degree angle so that the edge lines up with the bottom of the gum strip. Without licking it, fold the gum strip down over the folded corner and run your finger along it to make a crease the full length of the paper. Fold back this crease slightly, lick the gum strip, and fold it back down so that it seals the folded corner.

4 Wait a couple of minutes for the gum to dry and then open the paper out. You should have something resembling a cone.

5 Add some smoking mix to the cone (use a pencil to gently push the mix right into the tip) and pack it down so that the bottom third is filled, approximately 1½in (4cm). Now take a marker pen, approximately ⅝in (15mm) in diameter with a flat end, and one or two gum strips cut from rolling papers. Push the flat end of the marker into the top of the smoking mix and pinch the paper around the marker as if you were making a Dutch Tulip. Wrap the gum strips around the paper-encased marker, at the point where the marker meets the smoking mix.

6 Remove the marker and use your fingers to open and uncrease any of the paper that has been crushed together in the previous step. Now fill the next third of the paper with smoking mix and pack it down so that it fills out the paper and forms a spherical shape. Insert the paper tube into the top of the smoking mix and pinch the remaining paper tightly around it.

7 Cut another one or two gum strips and use them to secure the tube in place. Give it a minute for any gum to dry and then it's ready to smoke!

Oompa-Loompa, doobie-dee-doo...
I've got Double Bubble for you!!

T-BAR

Bin your bling, lose the lowrider, and ditch your gold grills...
there's a new Pimp Daddy in town and its name is T-Bar.
This badass mofo will get any party jumping and have
everyone wanting to join you in this double dose of deluxe
dopeness! The best bit is that it can be kept and used
again and again!

1 Take two pieces of paper or thin card, approximately 6x2in (15x5cm). Roll them into two tubes, approximately the same diameter as a pencil but one slightly wider than the other. Seal them both with tape or rolling papers.

2 Use a sharp knife or scissors to cut a hole half way along the wider tube. The other tube will need to fit snugly into this hole, so be careful not to cut the hole too big. It is a good idea to start small and gradually increase the size of the hole until it is just right.

3 Insert the narrower tube into the hole and seal the junction with tape or gum strips removed from rolling papers.

4 All that is left now is to roll two juicy joints, push them into each end of the T-Bar, and you'll soon have the party chanting your name like a true cheeba champion!

DEVIL'S TRIDENT

This menacing pitchfork of a spliff is known as a "Devil's Trident" because in order to survive one of these you will need to sell your soul to the devil! So get out your Ouija board, sacrifice a goat, and get ready for Beelzebub himself to appear in a flash of red smoke. Once you've parted ways with your eternal soul and put a Trident together, make sure Lucifer has a toke before he heads back down to Hell. Hopefully, you'll both forget why he came up to visit you in the first place!

1 Take two pieces of paper or thin card, one approximately 4x1½in (10x4cm) and the other 6x1½in (15x4cm). Roll them into tubes, making the shorter one slightly narrower than the other. Bear in mind that the longer tube needs to be a suitable diameter to insert a joint snugly into the end of it. Also, the shorter tube needs to be narrow enough to pass through the longer tube. Seal with tape or rolling papers.

2 Using a sharp knife or scissors, cut a hole about ¹/₂-⁵/₈in (10-15mm) from each end of the shorter tube. These holes must only go through one side of the tube and not all the way through. They also need to be the right size for the roach end of a spliff to be inserted. Next cut a hole all the way through the middle of the tube.

3 Now cut a hole all the way through the longer tube, approximately ³/₄in (20mm) from one end. Pass the shorter tube through it so that the center hole of the shorter tube lines up with the center of the longer tube. Make sure that air can clearly pass through.

4 Seal any gaps around the junction using tape or rolling papers. Also seal the open ends of the shorter tube.

5 Insert joints into each of the three holes and invite two of your friends over to even up the numbers. Just be careful not to take someone's eye out whilst lighting up this bad boy!

MJÖLNIR

Named after Thor's very own hammer, this hard-hitting creation was forged straight from the flames of a Viking's furnace. As its name suggests, it'll hit you over the head and leave you seeing Norse gods flying through the sky for days. This thunderous big brother of the T-Bar is not for the faint-hearted and, once you've nailed it, you'll have Odin himself worshipping the ground you walk on.

1 To make this colossal creation you will need two pieces of paper or thin card, approximately 6in (15cm) wide: one should be about 8in (20cm) long; the other only needs to be about two-thirds as long (5in/12cm).

2 Take the longer piece and fold back about ½in (1cm) at one end.

3 Flip it over and fold back again. Repeat until you have made four folds to create a concertina effect.

4 Flatten it down and, using a sharp knife or a pair of scissors, cut out the middle section of the concertina.

5 Roll the remainder of the paper or card around this concertina so that it becomes enclosed within a tube. From one end of the tube the concertina of paper/card should look like an "M." This will prevent any smoking mixture from being knocked or sucked out of the tulip buds.

6 Seal this tube closed with tape or rolling papers and then roll and seal the other piece of paper or card into a slightly narrower tube.

7 Using the knife or scissors, cut a hole in the middle of the wider tube on the side that the top of the "M" touches. It needs to be just the right size for the narrower tube to fit into, so make sure you don't cut this hole too big. It is best to start small and gradually make it bigger if you need to.

8 Wrap tape or rolling papers around the join to make sure it is airtight. Then make two tulips (see page 92) and attach them to each end of the wider tube; you can use gum strips or tie with thread.

Master this force to be reckoned with and there'll be a place waiting for you in the halls of Valhalla.

THAT'S DOPE!

The size of the wider tube made here is perfect for a standard two-paper tulip, but it can be made even bigger to accommodate larger tulips— if you are feeling brave enough!

A LITTLE PAUSE

After all that rolling and smoking, you'll no doubt be feeling a little stoned. Here are a few words of weed wisdom to think about while you build up the motivation to roll another joint...

"I used to smoke marijuana. But I'll tell you something: I would only smoke it in the late evening. Oh, occasionally the early evening, but usually the late evening—or the mid-evening. Just the early evening, mid-evening, and late evening. Occasionally, early afternoon, early mid-afternoon, or perhaps the late-mid-afternoon. Oh, sometimes the early-mid-late-early morning... But never at dusk."

Steve Martin

"Dope will get you through times of no money better than money will get you through times of no dope."

*Freewheelin' Franklin,
The Fabulous Furry Freak
Brothers' Comics*

"When you smoke the herb, it reveals you to yourself."

Bob Marley

"The illegality of cannabis is outrageous, an impediment to full utilization of a drug which helps produce the serenity and insight, sensitivity and fellowship so desperately needed in this increasingly mad and dangerous world."

Carl Sagan

"THAT IS NOT A DRUG. IT'S A LEAF."
Arnold Schwarzenegger

"It really puzzles me to see marijuana connected with narcotics, dope, and all of that stuff. It is a thousand times better than whiskey. It is an assistant and a friend."

Louis Armstrong

"They lie about marijuana. Tell you pot-smoking makes you unmotivated. Lie! When you're high, you can do everything you normally do just as well—you just realize that it's not worth the fucking effort. There is a difference."

Bill Hicks

BLUNT

You've completed the merger! You've won the case! You've sealed the deal! It's time to savor the moment and take a second to look out across the vast empire that you've built. This calls for a cigar... but with a difference. Kick back and ask your butler to fetch one of your finest Havanas before packing it to the rafters with sticky skunk. Due to the size of some of the cigars available, you may need a millionaire's bank balance to afford the pile of weed required to fill it!

1 To make a blunt you will need either a cigar or cigarello—the fatter the better, as it will give more width to the blunt paper and allow for easier rolling. Although cigars are not particularly cheap, the more expensive and higher quality cigars will be made with higher grade tobacco leaves and ultimately lead to a superior blunt. Blunt wraps are available to buy, but they

don't come close to the real deal and are best avoided. If your cigar has a closed end this must first be removed using a cigar cutter or a sharp knife. If the cigar has a label, this must also be removed.

2 Soak a small towel in warm water and then ring it out with your hands until no more water drips out. You want it to be damp but not overly wet. Now wrap the towel around the cigar for a few moments to moisten and soften it. You can also hold the cigar over the steam from a kettle or simply give it a good lick! Moistening the cigar can be repeated as much as is needed throughout, in order to keep it soft and prevent cracking.

3 Using a very sharp knife, start at one end and carefully cut down the full length of the cigar.

4 Insert a needle, toothpick, or any other suitable instrument into the cut and slide out the tobacco filling. It is best to remove a small section at a time, starting from the bottom and working up, so as to avoid damaging the outer layers.

5 You will now have an empty cigar skin that can be laid out flat. Most cigars have an outer "wrapper" of a tobacco leaf wrapped around a thicker layer of reconstituted tobacco called a "binder." The binder is the part you want to keep, so, using your fingers, peel away the outer wrapper leaf.

6 Many blunt connoisseurs will insist that a true blunt should be made without a roach. It all comes down to personal preference and ultimately there is no right or wrong way to get stoned! However, using a roach will prevent the end becoming clogged with moisture and tar, and give you something to hold without getting your fingers burned. Despite the ongoing tobacco/no tobacco debate among joint smokers, most blunt tokers will agree that only pure weed or a weed-and-hash mix should be rolled up. However, a blunt can take quite a lot of filling so in hard-up times a little tobacco can be used.

7 Whereas joints are rolled by sliding the sides of the paper past each other to shape the mix and then using a tuck-and-roll technique, blunts aren't as workable and their size can be restrictive. Instead, the filling is pressed into place from above with your fingers and the blunt skin rolled and gently pressed to get the desired shape and density.

8 Once the weed is shaped sufficiently, use your thumb to tuck the front part of the blunt skin in behind the filling. Although there is no gummed strip, as on a rolling paper, lick along the inside of the flap, as you would with a rolling paper, and seal the blunt closed.

9 Finally, lick the blunt thoroughly all over to fully seal it, give it a tap and a poke, and leave for a few minutes to dry. If it is really wet, you can carefully run the flame from a lighter along the outside of the blunt to help it dry.

This is one for the special moments in life. Blaze up and blunt out. You deserve it!

HOLLOW JOINT

A joint with a hole in it! Why would anyone do such a thing? Well, because as masters of our art, we can. Like a stuntman driving a somersaulting motorbike off a cliff and landing on the tongue of a blue whale, it's difficult, it's impressive, and people will applaud us for it. Not that we love the spotlight but, as Reverends of Rolling, we need to give the world a little reminder of what we can do every now and then. Perfect this technique and you'll have those junior-jointers double taking at your mastery.

1 Cut a piece of paper to about the size of a king size rolling paper, approximately 4x2in (10x5cm). Roll it into a very narrow and tight cone and seal it together with sticky tape, making sure there are no sticky sections of tape facing outward.

2 Lay this on a king size rolling paper with a small gap next to the narrow end and roll it up as if it were a joint. Try to roll it as tightly as you can.

3 Fold back the small section of empty paper at the narrow end and seal it closed with a piece of a gum strip removed from another rolling paper. Test to make sure that the paper cone can slide out of the rolling paper sleeve, but there is no need to remove it fully.

4 Lay a king size rolling paper flat out with the gum strip facing up and toward you and add an extra-wide roach. Spread out a thin layer of finely ground smoking mix all over the paper but not either side of the roach (as shown). You may find that pure weed works better for this roll, but if you do use tobacco make sure it is also ground up very finely with no hard lumps or sharp pieces. Lay the paper cone on top of the bed of weed, leaving a gap of approximately ½in (1cm) next to the roach.

5 Carefully pick up the paper so that the weed wraps around the paper cone, with a layer remaining intact underneath it. You will probably need to sprinkle some more smoking mix on top to give a complete and consistent layer.

6 Now roll it just as you would a standard One-skin (see page 72), but trying to keep the weed in a complete layer around the cone. Once rolled, poke the weed down the gaps in the end of the joint with a narrow poker and top up with extra weed to bring it level with the end. Then slide the paper cone out from inside its rolling paper sleeve, making sure not to pull the rolling paper out with it.

7 Trim any excess paper with a pair of scissors and give it a tap.

Now all that is left to do is step back, take a bow, and soak up the adulation!

TWISTER

Alert the storm chasers, batten down the hatches, and put on your mac; there's a storm a-brewing! Once you get this joint rolled, you'll have a natural disaster on your hands. This windy wonder is made up of three Two-skin joints that are braided together to form a triple-twisted spliff that will leave a trail of destruction in its wake! We would advise you to tie down your stash before attempting this roll as the weather patterns in your bedroom might get a little turbulent.

1 Although it is possible to use single length papers for a Twister, for a truly impressive creation a bit of extra length is needed. Rip-style papers are perfect for this; however, joining two king size papers together works just as well. To do this, use the technique explained in the Two-skin (see page 78).

2 Add a roach to the left-hand end of the paper and then add your smoking mix. Use your fingers to shape the mix into a fairly thin and even line.

3 Roll the joint fairly straight, even, and narrow. Due to the length you may want to rest one end on a raised surface while you work on the other end. If you are struggling to do this by hand, try using the Card Trick method (see page 127) but, instead of holding the paper in your hand, lay it down on a hard surface and use a ruler instead of a credit card. Alternatively, you could use a rolling mat. Tap the joint gently on a hard surface and give it a slight poke but do not twist it closed.

4 Roll two more joints in the same way, trying to make them as similar to each other as possible. Lay them out, side by side with the roaches lined up. Cut off the gum strips from two or three rolling papers and use them to bind the roach ends of the three joints together. Leave for a minute or two so that the gum strips are fully dry.

5 Take the joint from one side and pass it over the top of the middle joint so that they are snugly fitting together at the roach end. Then take the third joint and pass this over the one that is now in the middle. Again make sure they are fitting snugly together.

6 Now move the joint at the top of the diagram over the top of the joint that is now in the middle. Repeat this process of alternately folding the outside joints over the top of the middle joint, making sure at each stage that they are fitting together as closely as possible.

7 Once you have braided the full length of the joint, twist the three ends together and get ready to be blown away!

SCORPION

WARNING: this is a highly dangerous animal!
Handle with care!

This is Mother Nature at her finest. Roll this chronic creepy
crawly and you won't know whether to smoke him or put him in
a cage. To put it bluntly: this is one
huge joint with three smaller
ones pushed through to
create the legs and two
bigger ones for the arms;
both topped off with tulip bud
pincers... Get comfy, ladies
and gentlemen, because
this may a take
a while.

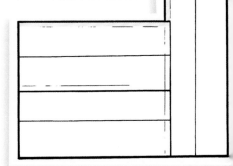

1 To make the body of the Scorpion you will need four king size
rolling papers. Lick the gum strip of one paper and stick it to
the bottom edge of another
paper. Then turn a third
paper by 90-degrees and
stick its gum strip to the
right-hand edge of the first
two papers. Be sure only to
lick the area of gum strip that
will be covered by the first
two papers.

2 Fold up the bottom half of the lower horizontal paper and crease all the way along, through the vertical paper. Lick this crease and tear off the bottom part of the papers. Then take the fourth paper and stick its gum strip to the right-hand edge of the third paper, again only licking the section of gum strip that will be covered up.

3 Add a roach, plenty of smoking mix, and roll the joint as you would a Three-skin (see page 86) but with a second flap. Tap and poke the joint but not overly so, as some flexibility will be needed later.

4 Next, get five more king size rolling papers. Roll two cone shaped One-skin joints (see page 72) but without roaches and roll the other three papers into skinnier straight joints, also with no roaches. Twist both ends of the skinny joints but leave both ends of the cones open. Take a needle or other sharp pointed instrument and make a small hole (big enough for air to pass through) all the way through the center of the three skinny joints.

5 We now need to make two mini Dutch Tulip buds (see page 92), so take two more king size papers and stick the gum strip of one to the bottom edge of the other. Lick along the center crease line of the lower paper, tear off the bottom section, and discard it. Now cut vertically through the center of the papers, splitting them in two.

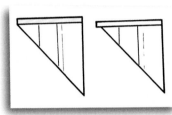

6 Fold the bottom left corner up at a 45-degree angle so that the edge lines up with the bottom of the gum strip. Without licking it, fold the gum strip down over the folded corner and run your finger along it to make a crease the full length of the paper. Fold back this crease slightly, lick the gum strip, and fold it back down so that it seals the folded corner. Repeat for the other section of rolling papers.

7 Cut or tear away the top part of both papers, as shown, so that the openings of the flattened tulip buds are level.

8 Open up these tulip buds and fill them with smoking mix, making sure to get it right in to the tips. Insert the conical joints (see step 4) into the tops of the smoking mix and pinch the paper around the stems of the joints to create the bud shapes. Secure the buds in place using the gum strips cut from a couple of extra rolling papers.

9 Using the needle again, poke a hole all the way through the center of the large joint.

10 Insert one of the skinny joints through this hole so that the hole in the center of the skinny joint lines up with the air channel of the large joint. Repeat for the two remaining skinny joints, making holes approximately ⅝in (15mm) apart from each other, moving toward the wider end of the large joint. Seal any gaps around these three joints with some more gum strips.

11 Make a fourth hole all the way through the large joint, this time a little further along than the spacing between the first three skinny joints, approximately ¾in (20mm). Insert the two mini Dutch Tulips into these holes and secure firmly with gum strips.

12 Gently bend the skinny joints down to form the legs, bend the tulip stems round and up slightly to make the arms, and finally bend the roach end of the large joint upward to make the scorpion's curled tail. It's best not to light all the joints at once; stagger them by first lighting the pincers, followed by the head, and finally the legs.

Now, get ready because one sting from this critter's tail and you will be delirious for days.

TECHNICOLOR DREAM SMOKE

Bring together two colored papers to create an eye-catching joint like no other! Mix and match until you find the right color scheme for any occasion, whether it's peacocking at a party or supporting your favorite team.

1 Take two different colored rolling papers and flatten them out with their gum strips facing up and toward you.

2 Cut away the bottom of one paper at an angle, then lick the gum strip of the uncut paper and stick it along the bottom cut edge of the first paper.

3 Using a sharp knife or scissors, cut away the bottom and right sides of the lower paper so that it is the same size and shape as an uncut king size rolling paper.

4 Fold the paper horizontally along the center to make a new crease line, unfold it, and lay it out as you would a standard joint with the gum still facing upward and toward you. Add a roach and your smoking mix.

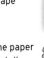

5 Finally roll it in the same way as you would a One-skin (see page 72).

Smoke this and you'll feel like you've found the pot o' gold at the end of a rainbow!

CARD TRICK

Any credit card, playing card, ruler, or rolling paper packet can be put to good use in making a tightly rolled spliff. Magic!

1 Begin by preparing a rolling paper as you would for a standard One-skin with a roach and your smoking mix. As with a One-skin, slide the back and front parts of the rolling paper back and forth past each other to shape the smoking mix inside into the desired baseball bat shape.

2 Rather than using the tuck-and-roll technique, hold the paper in your left hand so that the center crease of the paper is resting on top of your middle finger, your index finger is running along the back edge of the paper, and your thumb is supporting the front.

3 Pick up a card in your right hand and push the bottom edge of it into the front of the rolling paper along the top edge of where the smoking mix is inside. Move it back and forth from left to right along the paper to compress the mix tightly into shape.

4 While moving the back-side of the paper up slightly with your index finger, push the card (and the front part of the paper) down tightly behind the smoking mix.

5 Once the full length of the paper is tucked in behind the mix, keep applying gentle pressure on the joint with the left hand to prevent it unrolling and slide out the card with your right hand. If you find that you also need to use your

right hand to hold the joint together, you can use your mouth to pull out the card. Now lick the gummed edge of the paper and use your thumbs to roll up the rest of the joint, sealing it closed. Give the joint a gentle tap on a hard surface, poke the end, and give it a twist.

– Part Three –
COOK IT
INTRODUCTION

You've successfully grown and harvested your first crop of sticky, sweet buds, and maybe even made some ultra-potent hash too, but what's the best way to enjoy the fruits of your labor? A key thing to consider is the temperature to which your cannabis is heated, because anywhere above 315°F (157°C) and you begin to lose cannabinoids (the good stuff). A joint can contain as little as 10 percent of the potential THC, while a bong will give you around 40 percent. A vaporizer is a better option, providing a potential THC hit of anywhere from 50 percent up to 95 percent, and without the harmful combustion by-products like carbon monoxide that you get with a joint or bong.

The Volcano vaporizer (right) is widely considered to be the best on the market, with superior build quality and exceptional performance. In all forms of smoking and vaporization, though, as much as 30–40 percent of the inhaled THC is lost when the vapor is exhaled.

WHY EAT YOUR WEED?

By far the healthiest and most efficient way to absorb cannabinoids is to eat or drink them, which ensures that 100 percent of them enter your body. However, the rate of absorption is much slower than when inhaled, usually taking 30–90 minutes to have an effect. The high also lasts considerably longer, with effects sometimes as long as ten hours. If you are unsure of the potency, eat a small amount and wait a couple hours before eating any more. If you do end up having a bad trip, try drinking the juice from fruits containing citric acid, such as orange or grapefruit, to reduce the effects. Eating pistachios or pine nuts can also help, as both contain pinene, a chemical that improves mental clarity.

Weed shouldn't just be eaten raw, as there are some properties that are brought on by heat. The THC present in raw weed is in its non-psychoactive form, tetrahydrocannabinolic acid (THCA). At 115–122°F (46–50°C) it begins releasing carbon dioxide and converts into its psychoactive form, tetrahydrocannabinol (THC). This reaction is known as decarboxylation.

To be readily absorbed by the body, cannabinoids must first be dissolved. As they are lipophilic (can be dissolved in fats and oils), people usually extract the cannabinoids into butter, vegetable oil, or milk. These can be used, even when cold, to make cannabis-infused food and drink, referred to as "edibles."

The cannabinoids are also soluble in alcohol, so "tinctures" can be made by extracting cannabinoids into drinks with a high alcohol content. However, cannabinoids are insoluble in water. This is why brewing cannabis tea is not very effective unless the drink is combined with milk.

One final point: the serving quantities provided are suggestions only and will vary depending on the strength of the canna butter/oil/milk and your personal tolerance levels. Go easy at first, it's better to use too little than too much.

HOW TO MAKE CANNA BUTTER AND OIL

Right, you must have developed quite an appetite with all the work you've put into growing your weed, so now it's time to cook up some tasty treats. The key ingredient to most cannabis-infused recipes is canna butter or oil, which can even be made from the trimmings left over from harvest.

You will need:

- 2–4oz (50–100g) weed trimmings or 1–2oz (25–50g) buds, dried and ground (quantities can be varied to suit personal preference)
- Baking tray
- Aluminum foil
- Oven thermometer
- Large pan
- 3 pints (1.5 liters) water
- 16oz (450g) butter or 2 pints (1 liter) vegetable oil
- Cheesecloth (muslin) and kitchen strainer (sieve)
- 2 large containers
- 4 tbsp soy lecithin powder/ granules (optional)

1 Before you make the canna butter, the THC in the weed must undergo a process called decarboxylation (see page 129). To do this, preheat the oven to 220-240°F (104-116°C/gas mark 1). Keep the temperature within this range and never let it exceed 300°F (150°C/gas mark 2). Spread the weed out on a baking tray and cover with foil, loosely but sealed tightly around the tray. Put into the oven for 30 minutes. Leave to cool fully before opening the foil, to prevent vapor loss.

2 Heat up the water in the pan, add the butter or oil and weed, stir, and bring to the boil. Reduce to a very low heat, put the lid on, and simmer for 2-3 hours, stirring occasionally.

3 Fold the cheesecloth (muslin) into a double layer, place in the strainer (sieve) and put that into a large container. Pour the mixture through.

4 Once all the liquid has drained through, bundle up the wet weed inside the cheesecloth and squeeze out as much remaining liquid as possible.

5 If using butter, put the container into the refrigerator. After a while the water and butter will separate, with a layer of butter solidifying on top of the water. Once separated, discard the water.

If using oil, leave the mixture out for 1-2 hours so the oil and water separate. Then put it in the freezer for 4-6 hours so the water freezes and you can pour off the oil. If the oil has coagulated in the freezer, scrape it off. It will liquefy at room temperature.

6 The butter or oil can be used as it is, but it can be further improved with the introduction of lecithin. When added, it will make the effects of the cannabis come on much faster and feel a lot stronger. Gently melt or warm the canna butter or oil in a pan, stir in the lecithin until it dissolves, then pour the butter or oil back into the storage container. This will keep for about a month, or longer if frozen. Use it in place of some, or all, of the butter or oil in any recipes.

TO MAKE CANNA MILK

Replace the butter or oil with milk and don't add water. As no water has been added, no subsequent separation is required.

WAKE AND BAKE BANANA PANCAKES

Wakey, wakey! Rise and shine! It's a beautiful day you're missing out on! What's that? Your head's a bit groggy? I'm not surprised, with the amount of weed you smoked last night! Never fear, I've got just the thing for you: Wake and Bake Banana Pancakes! They're the tasty way of getting your breakfast buzz back on. These are small, American-style pancakes made with nutritious bananas and a generous helping of canna milk to set you up for the day!

Method

1 In a mixing bowl, mash up the banana with a fork really well so it becomes a smooth paste.

2 Sift the flour and baking powder into the bowl.

3 Add the egg, milk, and melted butter, if using. Thoroughly mix, using an electric mixer if possible, so that it becomes creamy and aerated. For oaty pancakes you can swap some of the flour with an equal quantity of oatmeal.

4 Warm a frying pan over a medium heat. When sufficiently hot, melt a little butter in the pan. Then spoon or pour in enough batter to make a pancake about 4in (10cm) wide. Fill up any more space in the pan with pancakes, being careful not to let them spread into each other.

Ingredients

- 1 over-ripe banana
- 1 cup (4oz/120g) all-purpose (plain) flour
- 1 tsp baking powder
- 1 egg
- ¼ pint (140ml) canna milk
- 1oz (25g) butter or canna butter, melted (optional)
- Butter, for frying

Makes 12 pancakes

5 When bubbles start appearing on the surface of a pancake, flip it over with a spatula and cook for another minute or so on the other side.

6 When sufficiently cooked on both sides, remove from the pan and carry on cooking more pancakes with the remaining batter.

7 Serve with maple syrup at breakfast time or enjoy with ice cream for a dank dessert!

CINNAMON DOPE-NUTS

You might think that cops and stoners don't have much in common, especially if you've ever had the misfortune of getting busted smoking or growing a bit of weed. Well, you're right for the most part, they don't usually see eye-to-eye, and cops should be avoided at all costs. However, one bond that we do share is a love for sweet and unhealthy food–especially donuts! So keep a stash of these handy, and if you're ever unlucky enough to have your rights read, offer some to the boys in blue and hopefully they'll soon be too baked to remember why they turned up in the first place.

Method

1 Preheat the oven to 350°F (180°C/ gas mark 4). Spray or grease two 6-hole donut pans well.

2 Sift the dry ingredients together into a large bowl. Melt the canna butter in another bowl in a microwave and then add the egg, milk, and vanilla. Then whisk it all together. Pour this mixture into the dry ingredients and stir until it's all combined.

3 Pour the batter into the donut pans so each hole is about three-quarters full. Bake in the oven for 15–20 minutes. They are ready when you poke them with a knife and it comes out clean.

4 While the dope-nuts are cooling, make the coating. Mix the sugar and cinnamon together in a bowl then melt the remaining butter in a pan. Now dunk each dope-nut in the melted butter and roll it in the sugar and cinnamon.

Ingredients

- 2 cups (9oz/250g) all-purpose (plain) flour
- 1½ cups (10½oz/300g) superfine (caster) sugar
- 2 tsp baking powder
- 1 tsp ground cinnamon
- ½ tsp ground nutmeg
- ½ tsp salt
- 1oz (30g) canna butter
- 1 large egg
- 10fl oz (300ml) full-fat (whole) milk
- 2 tsp vanilla extract

For the coating:

- ½ cup (3½oz/100g) sugar
- ½ tsp ground cinnamon
- 4oz (120g) canna butter

Makes 12 dope-nuts

PEANUT SHATTER

Be very, very careful... this is the most fragile cannabis confectionery you will ever eat. This nutty toffee treat pays homage to butane honey oil, also known as BHO or "shatter," the most potent type of hash there is. Not everyone can get their hands on real shatter, but with this recipe you can have the next best thing. So cook up a batch and handle with care, because both this delicate delicacy and your mind are about to get shattered!

Method

1 Grease or line a large baking sheet, preheat the oven to 400°F (200°C/gas mark 6), and put the sheet in fo warm.

2 Place the sugar, corn (golden) syrup, and water in a large pan and bring to a boil over a medium heat, stirring frequently so it doesn't burn.

3 Mix in the peanuts and heat until the temperature reaches 300°F (150°C). This will take about 15 minutes.

4 Remove the baking sheet from the oven.

5 Stir the canna butter into the toffee until it has melted. Remove from the heat and immediately mix in the baking powder.

6 Pour the mixture into the tray, spreading it all the way to the edges with two forks.

7 Leave to cool completely, at least 1 hour, before shattering into pieces ready to be devoured.

Ingredients

- 1½ cups (10½oz/300g) sugar
- 8fl oz (225ml) corn (golden) syrup
- 8fl oz (225ml) water
- 16oz (450g) honey-roasted peanuts (or any other nuts)
- 3 tbsp canna butter
- 1½ tsp baking powder
- Cooking/candy thermometer

Serves 6–10

CARAMEL AND CASHEW CANNA COOKIES

Forget "more-ish," these cookies are downright addictive! They're so alluringly packed with the perfect pairing of salted cashew nuts and sticky caramel pieces, you won't be able to put the cookie jar down. Just be careful that one bite doesn't lead to you scoffing the whole lot, though, as they are loaded with potent canna butter and will leave you more baked than the inside of your oven. These irresistible edibles are definitely not the best idea for your work coffee breaks!

Method

1 Preheat the oven to 350°F (180°C/gas mark 4) and grease or line two large baking sheets.

2 Roughly break up the cashew nuts.

3 In a mixing bowl, cream together the butter and sugars.

4 In a separate bowl, lightly beat the egg. Add to the creamed butter and sugar along with the vanilla and mix together.

5 Sift in the flour, salt, and bicarbonate of soda and mix together.

6 Add the chopped caramels and cashew nuts to the dough and mix in.

7 Roll the dough into balls about 2in (5cm) wide and flatten slightly onto the baking sheets. Don't pack the cookies in too close together as they do spread out a lot when cooking.

8 Bake in the oven for 8 minutes for a really gooey cookie or up to 14 minutes for a slightly crisper one. They may seem undercooked, but they will harden considerably as they cool.

Ingredients

- 3½oz (100g) salted cashews
- 3½oz (100g) caramels. If you can't get caramel pieces, cut up some larger caramel candies or even slice up chocolate-coated caramel bars.
- 4oz (125g) softened canna butter
- ½ cup (3½oz/100g) soft light brown sugar
- ½ cup (3½oz/100g) superfine (caster) sugar
- 1 egg
- 1 tsp vanilla extract
- 1¾ cups (8oz/225g) all-purpose (plain) flour
- 2 tsp salt
- ½ tsp bicarbonate of soda

Makes 12–18 cookies

CARAMEL PECAN POT-CORN

We're off to the movies! Ever since the release of the unintentionally hilarious anti-weed film *Reefer Madness* in 1936, cannabis culture and cinema have gone hand in hand. The ground-breaking *Easy Rider*, smoking Labrador with Cheech and Chong, rolling a Camberwell Carrot in *Withnail & I*, f***ing up the rotation with Smokey in *Friday*, the Dude in *The Big Lebowski*, the back of a twenty-dollar bill (...on weed!) in *Half Baked*, getting the munchies for White Castle with *Harold & Kumar*, and cross-joints of *Pineapple Express*... and what better way to enjoy these canna classics than by rolling a fat joint of home-grown and tucking into a bowl of sticky, nutty, pot-laden popcorn!

Method

1 In a large pan, heat the vegetable oil and add the popcorn kernels. Put a lid on the pan and cook for 3–4 minutes. Shake the pan occasionally until the popping stops and then transfer to a large bowl.

2 Wipe the pan clean with a cloth. Dice the canna butter and add it to the pan along with the sugar and honey. Heat gently, stirring all the time, until the sugar has completely dissolved.

3 Bring to the boil and bubble rapidly, without stirring, for 4–5 minutes. The mixture will be ready when it has turned a caramel color.

4 Add the popcorn and chopped pecans and thoroughly stir until all the popcorn is coated in caramel and nuts.

5 Empty the pan onto a couple of non-stick baking sheets and leave to cool. Once cooled and hardened, break up into pieces and serve in a bowl.

Ingredients

- 2 tbsp vegetable oil
- 7oz (200g) popcorn kernels
- 4oz (125g) canna butter
- ¾ cup (5oz/150g) superfine (caster) sugar
- 2 tbsp clear honey
- ¾ cup (3½oz/100g) chopped pecans

Serves 2–4

'MALLOW BROWNIES

No weed cookbook would be complete without a brownie. The originator of all the culinary cannabis creations that have been concocted since, it deservedly earns its place in the history books as well as the cookbooks. But with the brownie well into its golden years, it's the perfect time to give it a bit of a makeover. So, what better way to make the stoner's favorite even greater than by topping it with melted marshmallows and more chocolate!

Method

1 Preheat the oven to 350°F (180°C/ gas mark 4) and line or grease a 9x13in (23x33cm) baking tray.

2 In a large bowl, cream together the sugar, butter, cocoa powder, and vanilla.

3 In a separate bowl, lightly beat the eggs and add to the mixture. Sift in the flour and baking powder and mix thoroughly.

4 When mixed, stir in the white chocolate chunks. Make the chunks reasonably large so they don't melt away in the oven.

5 Pour the mixture into the prepared tray, spreading it all the way into the corners. Bake in the oven for 25–30 minutes, until the top looks cooked.

6 Remove from the oven and cover the top of the brownie with a blanket of marshmallows, then sprinkle the chocolate chips on top.

7 Return to the oven for a few minutes so the marshmallows melt slightly and begin to turn brown.

8 It will be really hot and sticky, so resist the temptation to dive straight in; instead leave it to cool fully before taking out of the tray and cutting into pieces.

Ingredients

- 2 cups (14oz/400g) sugar
- 8oz (225g) canna butter, melted
- 2½oz (60g) unsweetened cocoa powder
- 1 tsp vanilla extract
- 4 eggs
- 1¾ cups (8oz/225g) all-purpose (plain) flour
- ½ tsp baking powder
- ½ cup (3½oz/100g) white chocolate chunks
- 7oz (200g) mini white marshmallows
- ½ cup (3½oz/100g) milk chocolate chips

Makes 18 brownies

RASTA PASTA

Put on a Bob Marley album, light up the chalice, and "pass the kouchie pon de left hand side," because it's time to pay homage to the Rastafari movement, a way of life that has become synonymous with weed and cannabis culture. This recipe fuses Italian and Jamaican influences by combining cheesy pasta with jerk chicken. Red peppers, green peppers, and golden corn are added to represent the famous Rasta colors, then of course the all-important ingredient– plenty of ganja to make you feel irie!

Method

1 Put all the marinade ingredients into a food processor and blitz until smooth. Place the chopped chicken breasts in a dish and smother with the marinade. Cover with plastic wrap (cling film)and refrigerate for at least an hour (overnight if you can wait that long).

2 Bring a large pan of water to a boil (this will be for the pasta). Meanwhile, melt the butter in another pan, add the flour, and stir until it forms a smooth paste. Then pour in the milk, stirring well with a hand whisk.

3 Put the marinated chicken into a frying pan and cook over a medium heat until browned. Add the chopped peppers and corn to the frying pan and continue to cook over a medium heat.

4 Tip the pasta into the boiling water and cook as per the packet's instructions.

5 Meanwhile, slowly bring the sauce to a boil, stirring continuously until it thickens. Remove the pan from the heat and stir in the cheese.

6 When the pasta is ready, the chicken is fully cooked, and the peppers are soft, drain the pasta and mix them all together, ready to be served.

For the jerk marinade:
- 5oz (150g) chopped onion
- 1 scotch bonnet or other chili, deseeded and chopped
- 1oz (30g) fresh ginger, peeled and chopped
- ½ tsp ground allspice
- A few sprigs fresh thyme, leaves only
- ½ tsp ground black pepper
- 3fl oz (75ml) white wine vinegar
- 3fl oz (75ml) dark soy sauce

- 4 chicken breasts, chopped
- 2oz (50g) butter (or canna butter for extra potency)
- ½ cup (2oz/50g) all-purpose (plain) flour
- 1 pint (500ml) canna milk
- 1 red bell pepper, chopped
- 1 green bell pepper, chopped
- 3½oz (100g) canned corn kernels
- 10oz (300g) pasta
- 4oz (120g) grated cheese

Serves 4

STONED BAKED PIZZA

You've heard of the Leaning Tower of Pisa, but what about the "lean power of pizza"?! Well, when it comes to food that gets you high, this Italian-inspired snack can't be topped. This is the perfect party food for slicing up and sharing with hungry stoner friends, and as both the base and the sauce are made using potent canna oil, it's probably a good thing if you don't scoff it all by yourself!

For the sauce:

- 14oz (400g) canned chopped plum tomatoes
- 3 tbsp tomato paste
- 3½fl oz (100ml) canna oil
- 2 garlic cloves, minced
- ½ tbsp dried basil
- ½ tbsp dried oregano
- ½ tbsp chili powder
- ½ tsp salt
- ½ tsp ground black pepper

- 10fl oz (300ml) warm water
- 1 sachet fast-action dried yeast
- 1 tbsp sugar
- 3 tbsp canna oil
- 3 cups (13oz/375g) all-purpose (plain) flour, plus extra for dusting
- 1 tsp dried thyme
- 1 tsp salt
- 2 large handfuls grated mozzarella

Makes 2 pizzas

Method

1 Put all the sauce ingredients into a pan and cook over a medium heat, stirring well. Bring to a gentle boil, then lower the heat and simmer for 30 minutes, stirring occasionally. Remove from the heat, transfer to a bowl, and refrigerate for a couple hours before using.

2 To make the pizza base, mix the water, yeast, sugar, and oil in a bowl. Add the flour, thyme, and salt. Mix and knead for 10–12 minutes, sprinkling with flour to stop it sticking to the bowl.

3 The dough should be elastic and smooth. Place it in an oiled bowl, drizzle with some more oil, cover with plastic wrap (cling film), and leave to stand for an hour.

4 Separate the dough into two halves and roll them into balls. Cover with a damp dish towel and leave to stand for another 10 minutes. Preheat the oven to 400°F (200°C/gas mark 6).

5 Roll the dough out onto two pizza pans or stones and poke some holes in it with a fork to let steam escape while cooking. Now all that's left is to smother your pizza bases with the special tomato sauce, sprinkle on some grated mozzarella cheese, and add any of your favorite toppings, if you like. Bake in the oven for about 20 minutes.

GROOVY SMOOTHIES AND HAZY SHAKES

After all this cooking in a hot kitchen you've no doubt got a thirst to quench. Luckily canna cooking isn't just limited to candy, cakes, and dinners; by brewing up a batch of weed-infused milk (see page 131) you can make refreshing shakes and smoothies. They're perfect for washing down some other THC treats or soothing your throat after a big bong hit. If you're after a health kick, the smoothies both contain two of your five fruit or veg a day, and surely the weed counts as a third one... doesn't it?!

Method

To make these delicious drinks, simply whizz all the ingredients together in a blender. Each one will serve two people.

Banana, Kiwi, and Ginger Smoothie

- 9fl oz (250ml) canna milk
- 1 banana, peeled and sliced
- 1 kiwi fruit
- Handful of ice
- 1 tbsp honey
- 1 tsp vanilla extract
- 1in (2.5cm) piece finely grated ginger

Strawberry and Cinnamon Smoothie

- 9fl oz (250ml) canna milk
- 1 banana
- 5 strawberries
- handful of ice
- 1–2 tsp ground cinnamon

Quadruple Chocolate Milkshake

- 9fl oz (250ml) canna milk
- 2 tbsp chocolate syrup
- 1 tbsp unsweetened cocoa powder
- 1 pint (500ml) chocolate ice cream
- Your favorite chocolate bar, chopped into pieces

Cookies and Cream Milkshake

- 9fl oz (250ml) canna milk
- 1 pint (500ml) vanilla ice cream
- 1 tsp vanilla extract
- 8 Oreo cookies, broken into pieces

GANJA GUACAMOLE AND SKUNK SALSA

Hola amigos! It's time to turn the heat up in here and get a bit spicy! From Mexican Rudy and Acapulco Gold to Cheech and Chong, "La Cucaracha," and even the word "marihuana," Mexico and cannabis have a long history together. So don't siesta, let's fiesta by piling up some tortilla chips and smothering them in Skunk Salsa and Ganja Guacamole, plus a dash of sour cream and some sliced jalapeño peppers to finish it off.

Ganja Guacamole

- 3 ripe avocados, halved, with stones removed
- 1 ripe tomato, chopped
- 1 small red onion, finely chopped
- 1 chili, deseeded and finely chopped
- Handful of cilantro (coriander), chopped
- Juice of 1 lime
- 2 tbsp canna oil
- Salt and black pepper

Method

1 Scoop out the flesh of the avocados into a bowl, then add the tomato, onion, chili, and cilantro (coriander). Add the lime juice and canna oil, and season with salt and pepper.

2 Use a fork to mash it all up until it gets to your preferred consistency.

Skunk Salsa

- 4 ripe tomatoes, chopped
- ¼ red onion, chopped
- ¼ red bell pepper, chopped
- Handful of cilantro (coriander), chopped
- 3 garlic cloves, minced
- 1 jalapeño pepper, finely chopped
- Juice of 1 lime
- 4 tbsp canna oil
- Salt and black pepper

Method

Mix all the ingredients in a bowl and season with salt and pepper. Toss thoroughly and leave to stand for 30 minutes before serving.

INDEX

THANKS

Firstly, I would like to say a massive thanks to Pete for giving me the opportunity to write this book. It's been a lot of fun to write, even more fun making the joints (especially testing them!), and it's a privilege to be able to make a book that hopefully will be enjoyed by like-minded stoners around the world for many years to come. Also, thanks to Clare for editing, Paddy and Jerry for your design, and everyone else involved at Dog 'n' Bone Books.

A huge thank you as well to John for your inspired illustrations, I'm so pleased you were involved in the project; and to Phil for all your creative-writing help, you really saved the day.

I must say a special thanks to my mates Joe, Mehmet, Rat, and Adrian for being my smoking buddies all these years and for your help with this book (including all the testing!).

Some other people who deserve credit for making me the seasoned stoner and veteran roller that I am are: Sam (for having our first joints together all those years ago); Ben, Big Pete, Dave, Deano, Little Pete, Matt, and Mide (for three hazy years in Leeds); Will (for the one-flakes and everything else over the years); and Aydin (for the Starburst and everything else back in the day).

Also, shout outs to the following friends (hopefully they might buy a copy if their names are in this!): Christian, Gary, Mike, Robin, Steve, Sean, Savio, Amit, Willy, Natalie, and Justin.

Of course, I mustn't forget to mention my family: Mum and Dad; Tony, Chris, Helen, and Sarah; and finally James, Katie, Amelia, and Dominic (you have all this to look forward to one day!).

If I've forgotten anyone, I'm sorry, I love you too; but it's 3am, I'm pretty stoned, and I don't have your number in my phone!

D